About the Author

Elaine Magee, M.P.H., R.D. is a regular contributor to *Woman's Day*, *Parenting*, and *Family Fun* magazines with occasional features in *Cooking Light* and *Fitness* magazines. She is the author of more than twenty books, including *Tell Me What to Eat if I Have Diabetes*, *Tell Me What to Eat if I Have IBS*, *Tell Me What to Eat if I Have Acid Reflux*, *Eat Well for a Healthy Menopause*, and *The Recipe Doctor*. She also has a recipe column called The Recipe Doctor, which is syndicated by Knight Ridder Tribune Wire Service and appears in newspapers across the country. Magee lives with her family in California.

The Flax
COOKBOOK

❧

Recipes and Strategies
to Get the Most from the
Most Powerful Plant on the Planet

ELAINE MAGEE, M.P.H., R.D.

MARLOWE & COMPANY
NEW YORK

Library of Congress Control Number: 2002113808
ISBN 1-56924-507-X

9 8 7 6 5 4 3 2 1

Designed by Pauline Neuwirth, Neuwirth & Associates, Inc.

Printed in the United States of America
Distributed by Publishers Group West

This book is dedicated to my amazing and loving father, Don (1922–2002). Papa, your big heart, abundant creativity, and sheer joy of living are a constant inspiration to me. My heart is full with love and memories of you—now and always.

Contents

Introduction

THE CLOSEST THING TO A MAGIC BULLET

NINETY-NINE CENTS a pound. That's the price of what is arguably the most powerful plant food on the planet. Flaxseed isn't new—it's been around for centuries. It's not exotic—it's an amber-colored seed the size of a sesame seed. You don't even have to choke it down—it actually has a pleasant, nutty taste. Who says you can't get anything for a buck anymore?

Flaxseed must be nature's best-kept secret. Here's this wonderful plant food that boasts not one but three nutritional attributes—both types of fiber, plus phytoestrogens called lignans, and a plant form of omega-3 fatty acids—yet no one knows about it. Sure, some people have started hunting down flaxseed and adding it to their smoothies, hot oatmeal, and bread—but not many. All you have to do is ask the people around you. Your average person doesn't even know what flaxseed looks like, let alone that it offers an array of essential nutrients. Flaxseed wasn't even being studied by the scientific community until about a decade ago.

"**CURRENT** research supports several health benefits from eating flax seed including a lower risk of heart disease, cancer prevention, management of autoimmune disorders, and relief of constipation."

FLAX COUNCIL OF CANADA

I have spent the past few years writing the Tell Me What to Eat medical nutrition series (Career Press), covering everything from diet, menopause, and type 2 diabetes to eating to prevent breast and colon cancer. No matter which book I worked on, I kept coming across strong, accumulating scientific evidence about the benefits of this itty-bitty seed called "flax." Well, you don't have to hit me over the head more than once—it got my attention.

I'm not one to promote magic bullets; I'm a firm believer in looking at your food intake as a whole. But truly, if there were an "almost" panacea out there in Nutrition Land—this would be it. The scientific evidence only continues to accumulate on flaxseed and the momentum builds with each year of research. What is it about flax that makes it so magical?

THINKING OUTSIDE THE FLAXSEED BOX

ULTIMATELY THIS *IS* a flaxseed cookbook, so in addition to bombarding you with the latest information about flaxseed, I am also serving up an assortment of flaxseed recipes. Now, I fully expect that some of you will prefer the easier method of adding ground flaxseed to your smoothies, bread, and muffins—which works just as well. In fact, there are ample recipes to satisfy this preference in chapters 3, 4, and 5.

Others will be willing to push the flaxseed envelope and try flaxseed recipes for everything from appetizers to entrées and even desserts. If you are in this latter category, I hope you will feel that you have found the Promised Land of flax as you thumb through chapters 6, 7, 8, and 9.

While working on this book, my family came to expect flaxseed in almost everything I cooked up; any food that wasn't white as snow was suspect. But I still managed to surprise them quite often. When my girls drank their Mocha-ccino Freeze (page 72) and told me how much they liked it, I quickly made my flaxseed confession.

Fast Flax Overview

THE FLAX COOKBOOK goes into great detail about what's nutritious about flax, and what the scientific evidence is thus far, and provides 101 facts about flax and 85 recipes covering everything from appetizers to dessert. But here's a fast flax overview:

Flaxseed is an actual "seed" grown mainly in Canada and the Dakota states. It looks like a brown sesame seed. There is also a lighter color variety of flaxseed called golden flax. It has been around for thousands of years, and when ground (you need to grind it before you eat it, otherwise it passes through your system and you don't get all of its nutritional attributes) it looks a little like wheat germ, but has a nutty flavor.

There is much to report about flax's potential health benefits, based on the extensive studies that have already been conducted with rats and humans, with many more going on as you read this. The future looks bright for flaxseed. But many scientists are waiting for more evidence before officially recommending it.

At the level of 1 to 2 tablespoons of ground flax a day, there don't appear to be any negative health consequences to flaxseed consumption, and there are potentially many benefits. These include:

➤ Possible cancer prevention and reduction of tumor growth (such as breast, prostate, and colon)

➤ Reduced risk of heart disease—studies suggest that flax lowers the risk of blood clots and stroke, and cardiac arrhythmias, along with lowering total and LDL cholesterol and triglycerides, and even blood pressure

➤ Better regulation of bowel functions, and prevention of constipation

➤ Possible reduction of the blood glucose response to carbohydrates

➤ Possible benefits in many "hyper-stimulated" immune system diseases, such as rheumatoid arthritis

➤ Possible relief of breast pain related to a woman's hormone cycle (cyclical mastalgia)

When my husband raved about the Stuffed Red Bell Peppers (page 154) he had just stuffed himself with, I couldn't help but delight in telling him that they were full of flax.

WHAT'S THE IDEAL DAILY DOSE OF FLAX?

"ONE TABLESPOON OF ground flaxseed per day may provide some health benefits in some cases and is most likely safe," says Dr. Lilian Thompson of the University of Toronto, one of the first pioneers in flaxseed research. Dr. Thompson urges certain groups of people, including children, young adults, and women who are breast-feeding, pregnant, or trying to conceive to be cautious about consuming large amounts of flax. She considers 3 to 5 tablespoons a day to be a large amount and suggests a daily dose of 1 tablespoon instead.

Health Canada (Canadian Health and Welfare) recommends a daily omega-3 fatty acid intake of at least 0.5 percent of total calories. For people eating around 2,000 calories a day, this translates into about 1 gram of omega-3 fatty acids per day. (The United States, by the way, hasn't made any recommendations on omega-3 fatty acid intake yet.) One tablespoon of ground flaxseed provides about 1.5 grams of plant omega-3s (alpha-linolenic acid or ALA).

WHO SHOULD SHY AWAY FROM FLAX?

UNTIL MORE STUDIES on humans are completed, Dr. Thompson definitely recommends that certain groups of people not eat flax, including pregnant women and breast cancer patients taking tamoxifen or other breast cancer drugs. She advises this because we still do not have data on whether flaxseed lignans antagonize the action of tamoxifen.

MORE THAN JUST NUMBERS — THE RECIPE NUTRITION ANALYSIS

EACH RECIPE IN this book comes complete with a nutrient analysis covering obvious items such as calories; grams of protein, carbohydrate, and fat; milligrams of cholesterol and sodium; and grams of fiber. But since all fat is not created equal, each recipe also lists the grams of each "type" of fat: saturated, monounsaturated, and polyunsaturated. I used the ESHA Food Processor II database (Elizabeth Stuart Hands and Associates) to calculate all of the analyses. Now, don't get upset if these numbers don't add up perfectly to the total grams of fat; the difference could be due to the unnamed trans fat content.

Each recipe also notes the Weight Watchers Winning Points per serving. The only problem I found with their slide rule point estimator is that it only goes up to 4 grams of fiber and many of the recipes in this book have far more than that. Also note that some of these recipes are a little higher in fat than you might expect, but keep in mind that each tablespoon of ground flaxseed adds almost 3 grams of fat into the equation.

Lastly—and I'm super-excited about this—each recipe also includes the grams of omega-3 fatty acids and the grams of omega-6 fatty acids per serving. This information is vital to the flaxseed cause. You see, it would be rather senseless to add flaxseed to recipes that were swimming in omega-6 fatty acids—the few flaxseed omega-3s would be a drop in the omega-6 bucket, so to speak. Most of the recipes in this book contain more omega-3s than omega-6s, which is a really good thing in a country that consumes around twenty times more omega-6s than omega-3s, when it should be more like two to four times more.

If I could tell someone interested in eating healthily to do only a few things, adding ground flaxseed would be right up there along with eating five cups servings of fruits and vegetables a day, eating more fish and beans, eating a moderate low-fat diet, and switching to canola and olive oil when possible. After reading the arguments for flaxseed in chapter 1, I hope you'll see why I felt I had to write this cookbook.

1

The Convincing Case
for Flaxseed

*I*T WOULD SURE make my job easier if each of the various components of flaxseed were neatly related to its own health benefit. Then I could break down the components and show you the research for each component—for example, how the omega-3s help with heart disease while the lignans in flaxseed (phytoestrogens) help with cancer. But it isn't that simple; there are countless overlaps.

Lignans are tied to helping the immune system, but so are the omega-3s, just through different metabolic pathways. Lignans appear to offer a measure of protection against some cancers, but so do omega-3s—again through different mechanisms. And don't get me started on heart disease.

So, first I thought I would go over the nutritional components in flaxseed so you can find out what's really in this tiny seed. Then, so you can see for yourself what all this fuss is about, I will review the scientific research on three of the major components in flaxseed:

- ❖ lignans (phytoestrogens)
- ❖ alpha-linolenic acid (a plant omega-3 fatty acid), and
- ❖ fiber (soluble and insoluble)

To make sure all the flaxseed bases are being covered, I will then list some of the evidence gathered so far for flaxseed, according to the various disease benefits. So get ready—this is going to be one interesting ride!

If Flax Had a Nutrition Label

WHEN I STARTED researching flaxseed, I read all sorts of statements about what's in flax, for example, "Flax is about 40 percent oil, more than half of which is a plant form of the omega-3 fatty acid (ALA or alpha-linolenic acid)," and "Flaxseed contains more ALA than canola or soybean oil," and "Flax has just as much soluble fiber as oat bran." But I'm going to do what I tell inquiring consumers to do: when all else fails, check the nutrition information label to know for sure what's in there. Generally, these labels don't lie.

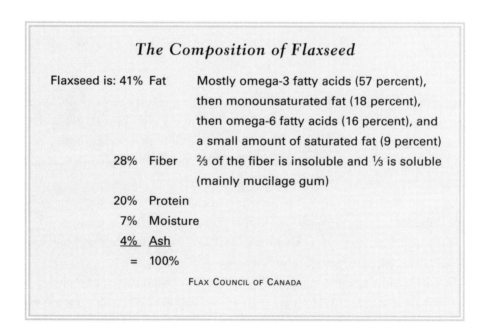

The Composition of Flaxseed

Flaxseed is:	41%	Fat	Mostly omega-3 fatty acids (57 percent), then monounsaturated fat (18 percent), then omega-6 fatty acids (16 percent), and a small amount of saturated fat (9 percent)
	28%	Fiber	⅔ of the fiber is insoluble and ⅓ is soluble (mainly mucilage gum)
	20%	Protein	
	7%	Moisture	
	4%	Ash	
	=	100%	

FLAX COUNCIL OF CANADA

The closest thing I could find to a nutrition information label for flaxseed was an itemized printout of all the specific nutrients in a tablespoon of flaxseed from the ESHA Research database. If we were to make a super-deluxe nutrition information label for ground flaxseed, this is what it would look like:

Ground Flaxseed

Serving Size: 1 tablespoon (8.13 grams)

Calories = 40

Protein = 1.6 g

Carbohydrate = 2.8 g

Total Fat = 2.8 g

Saturated Fat = 0.3 g

Monounsaturated Fat = 0.6 g

Polyunsaturated Fat = 1.8 g

Cholesterol = 0 mg

Total Fiber = 2.3 g

Sodium = 3 mg

Omega-3 fatty acids = 1.5 g

Omega-6 fatty acids = 0.3 g

<u>Vitamins and minerals</u>

Vitamin B6 = 6% RDA

Vitamin E = 6% DV

Folic Acid = 15% DV

Iron = 4% DV

Magnesium = 12.5% DV

Phosphorus = 6% DV

LET'S COMPARE

NO MATTER HOW you slice it, flaxseed is a food supplement. This means we aren't likely to eat it all by itself as we would a nut, for example, and although its taste is pleasant, it isn't something we are likely going to crave or *really* enjoy eating, as we would, say, chocolate. We are most likely going to be mixing it in with other foods or hiding it in certain favorite dishes, as we would oat bran or wheat germ.

Flaxseed operates like a grain in recipes, which begs the question: How does flaxseed compare nutritionally to oat bran and wheat germ? Of the three, which one has the most omega-3 fatty acids, or soluble fiber, or even folic acid? I've compared the three foods on page 11, and noted in boldface the amount of a particular healthful nutrient contained in that food that contains the most of it. I've got to warn you though: Flaxseed wins most of the categories, hands down.

There is one little catch. Different nutrition package labels and databases say a tablespoon of ground flaxseed weighs different amounts. One label said 2 tablespoons of ground flax weighed 13 grams, while a database computed 15 grams as 1 tablespoon of ground flax. What's a nutrition writer to do? I'm going to compare 15 grams each of flaxseed, oat bran, and wheat germ; please realize that this is around 2 tablespoons, give or take.

It only takes two weeks!

EAT a higher omega-3 diet for two weeks and you will already see a significant increase in desirable plant omega-3s (ALA) concentrations in body tissues (a three- to four-fold increase), according to an Australian study and earlier tudies by Stephen Cunnane, a researcher with the University of Toronto. At the same time, the less desirable omega-6 concentrations in the body tissues will be significantly decreased by the two-week mark.

ARGUMENT #1 — THE OMEGA CONNECTION

YOU CANNOT UNDERSTAND the health benefits of flaxseed without understanding the omega connection. You may have heard that omega-3 fatty acids are good for your heart and that we need to eat more fish because fish contain these omega-3 fatty acids. But that's just one big slice of the wonderful omega-3 pie. Some plant foods also contain a form of omega-3 fatty acids. And research has shown recently that plant omega-3s benefit the body in different ways than the fish omega-3s (more on this later in the chapter).

OMEGA-3s have been shown to modify several risk factors for coronary heart disease, including reducing serum triglycerides and blood pressure. They also protect against thrombosis and certain types of cancer, and modify immune and inflammatory reactions.

FLAX COUNCIL OF CANADA

SERVING SIZE: 15 GRAMS

	Flaxseed (about 2 Tbsp)	*Oat Bran* (about 2½ Tbsp)	*Wheat Germ* (about 2 Tbsp)
Calories =	**80.0**	37.0	54.0
Protein =	3.2 g	2.5	**3.5**
Carbohydrate =	5.6 g	**10**	7.7
Total Fat =	**5.4 g**	1.0	1.5
Saturated Fat =	**0.5 g**	0.2	0.25
Monounsaturated Fat =	**1.2 g**.	0.3	0.2
Polyunsaturated Fat =	**3.6 g**	0.4	0.9
Cholesterol =	0 mg	0	0
Sodium =	**6 mg**	0.6	0.4
Total Fiber =	**4.6 g**	2.3	2.0
Soluble Fiber=	**~1.5**	1	0.2
Insoluble Fiber=	**~3.0**	1.3	1.7
Omega-3 fatty acids =	**2.7 g**	0.03	0.12
Omega-6 fatty acids =	0.6 g	0.4	0.9
Omega-3 to Omega-6 ratio =	**4.2**	0.05	0.14

Vitamins and minerals (Percentage of Recommended Daily Allowance)

Vitamin B_6 =	**9%** DV	1.5%	6%
Vitamin E =	9% DV	3%	**27**%
Folic Acid =	**22%** DV	4.5%	21%
Iron =	6% DV	6%	6%
Magnesium =	**19%** DV	12%	12%
Phosphorus =	9% DV	13.5	**15%**

The Missing Link to the Omega Story

Here's the part of the story you may not have heard about. It isn't just important to work more high–omega-3 foods into our diet; we also need to *decrease* our omega-6 fatty acid foods. We should eat a ratio of up to four to one omega-6s to omega-3s, but in America, we are eating more like ten or twenty to one. That's a whole lot more omega-6s than we should be getting.

What happens when we eat far more omega-6s than omega-3s? The omega-6 fatty acids are metabolized, leading to the formation of compounds called eicosanoids that wreak havoc in your body. Too many of these omega-6s, which result in an excessive amount of eicosanoids,

- ❖ May help stimulate breast cancer growth and metastasis
- ❖ May be involved in blood clotting and may increase the risk of cardiovascular disease (although omega-6 metabolites are also involved in anti-clotting mechanisms as well)
- ❖ May not be good for the immune system

The bottom line: Not only do Americans desperately need to get more omega-3s into their daily diet, they also need to decrease their omega-6s.

Flaxseed to the Rescue

Flaxseed is one of the best plant sources of omega-3 fatty acids. It's about 40 percent oil, the majority of which (57 percent) is the plant form of an omega-3 fatty acid (alpha-linolenic acid, ALA). The oil from flaxseed actually contains more ALA than canola or soybean oil.

Your body can take this ALA, a short omega-3 fatty acid, and convert it into a long omega-3 fatty acid. Long omegas are more powerful in the body than short ones. We're encouraged to eat fish because omega-3 fatty acids in fish are the longer, more powerful type.

> ## Presto Chango—Some plant omega-3s turn into the long-chain omega-3s found in fish
>
> **ABOUT** 2 percent of plant omega-3s are converted to EPA (one of the long-chain omega-3 fatty acids found in fish) and about 0.5 percent are converted to DHA (the other long chain omega-3 found in fish). But there are things you can do in the rest of your diet to encourage this conversion as much as possible:
>
> ➤ Avoid eating a diet high in omega-6 fatty acids. A diet rich in omega-6s has been shown to reduce plant omega-3 conversion by as much as 40 percent.
>
> ➤ Avoid eating a diet high in saturated and trans-fatty acids. They also interfere with this desired conversion.

When you supplement your diet with a high omega-3 fatty acid food like flaxseed, you are helping to balance the omega-6 fatty acids in the typical American diet. Too much omega-6 fatty acid contributes to many of the chronic diseases in this country.

Today's Diseases and Omega Balance

Evidence of a link to omega imbalance is firm for some Western diseases and speculative for others. The following is a partial list of diseases that may be prevented or ameliorated with omega balance, in descending order of the strength of the available evidence:

1. Coronary heart disease and stroke
2. Essential fatty acid deficiency in infancy (i.e., affecting retinal and brain development)
3. Autoimmune disorders (i.e., lupus and nephropathy)
4. Crohn's disease
5. Cancers of the breast, colon, and prostate
6. Mild hypertension
7. Rheumatoid arthritis

There is almost instant gratification with omega balance—after three weeks on a high–omega-3 diet, research subjects have shown big differences in omega-6 levels in all body tissues. And in the secondary prevention of coronary heart disease, the effects of omega-3s appear to occur within the first four months of intervention.

Take Two Salmon and Call Me in the Morning

The omega-3 target set by many researchers can be met by including about four fatty fish meals per week, along with about 1½ teaspoons per day of a higher omega-3 oil. But most Americans aren't going to be able to sit down to fish four times a week and we would be hard-pressed to supply that much fish to all these people anyway, since about 60 percent of fish eaten in the U.S. is imported and many of the world's stocks are becoming depleted.

That's where flaxseed comes in—
It's an omega-3 plant source that
tastes good and is easy to eat every day

Why Balancing Omegas Is One of the Most Important Things You Can Do for Your Health

Balancing omegas is the missing piece to many disease puzzles. We are even feeding our commercial animals poorly—with high–omega-6 diets—and when we eat those animals and their products, we are feeding ourselves poorly, too. But just as we can manipulate animal feed to produce higher omega-3 eggs and chickens, we can also manipulate our own diets to keep our body tissues higher in omega-3s and lower in omega-6s.

Five Things You Need to Know about Omega-6 Fatty Acids

1. Omega-6 fatty acids are metabolized by the body, leading to the formation of many compounds, two of which may help stimulate breast cancer growth and metastasis.

2. Some of the omega-6 metabolites are involved in blood clotting; too much of them may increase the risk of cardiovascular disease. The omega-6, or arachidonic acid, is converted to thromboxane A_2 and eicosanoids, which tend to enhance atherosclerosis by promoting vasoconstriction and platelet aggregation, while omega-3 metabolites do the opposite.

3. Omega-6 metabolites affect the immune system and too much may not be good.

4. Metabolites from the omega-6, arachidonic acid, have been implicated in the development of certain clinical features of chronic inflammatory diseases such as systemic lupus erythematosus and rheumatoid arthritis.

5. If pregnant women have a high intake of omega-6s, the levels of the long–chain omega-3s found in fish (EPA and DHA) decrease in the umbilical plasma and therefore less of these omega-3s are getting to the developing baby.

Nine Things You Need to Know about Omega-3 Fatty Acids:

1. The North American diet is too high in total fat, saturated fat, omega-6 fatty acids, and trans-fatty acids and way too low in omega-3 fatty acids. This is a recipe for medical disaster.

2. Omega-3s appear to provide protection against:

   atherosclerosis and fatal cardiovascular events and strokes
   cardiac arrhythmias
   hypertension
   inflammatory disorders
   autoimmune disorders
   some types of cancer

3. Omega-3 fatty acids found in fish and some plant foods are metabolized into different compounds—which do not cause much of the inflammation and ill effects in the body that we see with the undesirable omega-6 metabolites.

4. In fact, when there is a large amount of these favorable omega-3s in the diet, they compete with the omega-6 fatty acids in the diet—reducing the undesirable omega-6 metabolites.

5. About 2 percent of plant omega-3s are converted to EPA and .5 percent to DHA (the long–chain omega-3s found in fish). A diet too high in omega-6s reduces this conversion by as much as 40 percent (The metabolization of omega-3s and omega-6s require the same enzymes so eating too much omega-6s will interfere with the metabolization of omega-3s.) Saturated fat and trans-fatty acids also interfere with the conversion of plant omega-3s to the more powerful omega-3s found in fish.

6. Substituting plant omega-3s for saturated fat in the diet enhances the blood cholesterol–lowering benefits of the omega-3s.

7. Omega-3s are considered essential for infant growth and development. Omega-3s, particularly DHA (an omega-3 found in fish), are required for nervous system and brain development and maturation of eyesight (visual acuity) in preterm and term infants. Health Canada recommends:

   Pregnant women consume an additional 0.05 grams of omega-3 fatty acids during the first trimester and an additional 0.16 grams during the second and third trimesters.

   Lactating women should increase their omega-3s by an additional 0.25 grams to benefit the developing baby, and also possibly to help lower the risk of postpartum depression.

8. Health Canada was the first to establish a recommended intake for omega-3s: 0.5 percent of total energy for omega-3 fatty acids as alpha-linolenic acid (the type of omega-3 found in plants).

9. When we feed our chickens a diet higher in omega-3s and lower omega-6s, we can produce eggs with seven to twelve times more omega-3s than regular eggs; one large egg can provide the same amount of omega-3s found in a three-ounce serving of fish. We can also produce chicken meat with far smaller amounts of omega-6 fatty acids per serving. Right now, because we feed chickens a high–omega-6 corn diet, the chicken we eat is fairly high in omega-6 fatty acids.

ARGUMENT #2 — THE HIGH-FIBER OPTION TO OAT BRAN

WE ALL KNOW that oat bran is a great source of soluble fiber, which helps lower blood cholesterol and normalize blood sugars. This cholesterol-lowering claim has been plastered on many a package of oats and oat cereals. A recent study from Mexico, in which researchers actually measured the effects of eating cookies enriched with oat bran, found that LDL ("bad" cholesterol) and plasma triglycerides were lowered after eight weeks in people with high blood cholesterol. Why not bake cookies pumped with nutty-tasting flaxseed instead? (By the way, there are several cookie recipes for you to try in chapter 9.)

Oat bran doesn't have the market cornered on soluble fiber. Tablespoon for tablespoon, **flaxseed actually contains more soluble and insoluble fiber than oat bran.**

> **INSOLUBLE FIBER** helps move things along in the intestinal tract and prevent constipation.
>
> **WATER-SOLUBLE** fiber helps maintain blood glucose levels and lower blood cholesterol levels.

Stephen Cunnane, Ph.D., a flaxseed researcher from the University of Toronto, studied what happens when women add about 2 tablespoons of ground flax to their daily diet for four weeks. Their total cholesterol fell 9 percent and their LDL ("bad") cholesterol dropped 18 percent; HDL ("good") cholesterol stayed the same. Similar results were also found in a different study conducted by researchers in the United States.

But the benefits of soluble fiber go beyond their link to serum cholesterol and heart disease. Soluble fiber helps people with diabetes normalize their blood sugar. Literally, the higher the fiber grams, particularly from soluble fiber–rich foods, the lower the blood sugars tend to be. This flaxseed bonus has a huge potential payoff, since type 2 diabetes continues to be an American epidemic, affecting over eighteen million Americans and counting. Soluble fiber also acts as an intestinal stabilizer, which comes in quite handy for the twenty-five to fifty-five million Americans who suffer from some degree of Irritable Bowel Syndrome — myself included.

Why Is Adding Fiber Such a Good Idea?

The definition of "fiber" is plant substances that we can't digest—so it moves through the entire intestinal tract and is eventually carried out of the body. How can something that we can't even digest and absorb be so good for us? Recently the American Dietetic Association (ADA) published a paper on fiber and noted that the recommended intakes of 20 to 35 grams per day for healthy adults and age-plus-5-grams per day for children (e.g., 15 grams for a ten-year-old) are simply not being met.

So should we all go out and pop a fiber pill? Absolutely not. According to the ADA, our ideal higher fiber foods—minimally processed fruits, vegetables, beans, and whole and high-fiber grain products—provide us with micronutrients and non-nutritive ingredients (such as plant estrogens and antioxidants) that are essential components of healthful diets, in addition to the fiber.

THE ADA says we should care about getting enough fiber because:

➤ Eating dietary fibers that are viscous (gummy and gelatinous) lowers blood cholesterol levels and helps to normalize blood glucose and insulin levels. This alone makes soluble fiber part of the dietary plans to treat cardiovascular disease and type 2 diabetes.

➤ Viscous soluble fiber interferes with bile acid absorption from the ileum (the lower end of the small intestines), which means less bile acid is getting reabsorbed and recycled. This causes more LDL or "bad" cholesterol to be removed from the blood and converted into new bile acids to replace the bile acids lost in the stool. There is even evidence that the presence of some viscous fibers in the intestines may decrease cholesterol synthesis—so you're getting cholesterol coming and going, so to speak.

Due to sufficient studies on certain types of soluble fiber, the FDA recently authorized a health claim that foods meeting specific compositional requirements and containing 0.75 to 1.7 grams of soluble fiber per serving can reduce the risk of heart disease.

Studies of people with type 2 diabetes suggest that high fiber diets reduce insulin demand. Two studies found that fiber from cereals, but not from fruits and vegetables, had an inverse independent relationship with risk of type 2 diabetes. This means that as intake of fiber from cereals and grains went up, the risk of type 2 diabetes tended to go down.

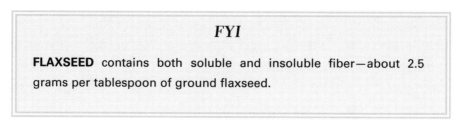

FYI

FLAXSEED contains both soluble and insoluble fiber—about 2.5 grams per tablespoon of ground flaxseed.

Flaxseed Provides Fiber That is Important for Many Reasons

❖ Fiber that is incompletely or slowly fermented by microflora (healthy bacteria) in the large intestine promotes normal bowel movements and is a vital component of diet plans to **treat constipation** and **prevent diverticulosis and diverticulitis**. A fiber-rich diet is also associated with a lower risk of colon cancer.

 I do caution you, though—generally, small seeds or husks that may not be fully digested in the upper gastrointestinal tracts are eliminated from the high-fiber diets of patients with diverticulosis, as a precaution against having these small pieces become lodged within a diverticulum (a small pocket in the intestines). This is another reason *not* to eat whole, unground flaxseeds. Flaxseeds have a pointy end, and this particularly may cause problems in an inflamed or irritated intestinal tract. Grinding your flaxseed or buying flaxmeal helps eliminate most of this risk.

❖ A fiber-rich meal is processed more slowly through the digestive tract, promoting earlier satisfaction, and is often less calorically dense and lower in fat and added sugars (all good for **weight loss and weight maintenance**)

❖ **Fiber may reduce the risk of colon and rectal cancers**. Recently, the results of thirteen case-control studies on diet and colorectal cancer rates were pooled and researchers concluded there was substantive evidence that eating fiber-rich foods is related to lowering risks of these cancers. The authors estimated that the risk of colorectal cancer in the U.S. population could be cut by about 31 percent by increasing high-fiber foods an average of 13 grams more fiber a day.

❖ **It is possible that fiber may also reduce the risk of breast cancer**.

Some studies have not found a relationship between fiber and breast cancer risk reduction, while others have. However, when researchers pooled the results of twelve case-control studies on dietary fiber and the risk of breast cancer, they found that a high fiber intake was associated with a reduced risk.

> **CAUTION**—All fiber intake recommendations need to recognize the importance of adequate fluid intake, and caution should be used when recommending fiber to those with gastrointestinal diseases, including constipation.

ARGUMENT #3 — FLAXSEED IS THE RICHEST SOURCE OF LIGNANS (PHYTOESTROGENS)

NO OTHER PLANT food even comes close to matching the lignan might of flaxseed. Flaxseed contains, by weight, over 120 times more lignan than most beans, over 180 times more lignan than most whole grains and cereals, and over 260 times more lignan than most fruits and vegetables. Let me explain to you why this is an amazing thing. Lignans are phytoestrogens (plant estrogens) that have weak estrogen activity in animals. They can interfere with estrogen metabolism in animals and humans. Some researchers now believe that these phytoestrogens can exhibit both estrogen and antiestrogen activity.

Lignans have several biological characteristics going for them. They are known to act as an:

❖ Antimitotic (discouraging a type of undesirable cell division)
❖ Antifungal (destroying or inhibiting the growth of fungi)
❖ Antioxidant (preventing or inhibiting undesirable oxidation)

Lignans have also been shown to:
❖ suppress the differentiation and growth of cultured human leukemic cells, possibly by interfering with DNA, RNA, and/or protein synthesis
❖ have a low potential to become toxic or damaging to normal immune cells.

What Does Our Body Do with Lignans Once We Eat Them?

WE eat the plant lignans in flaxseed—SDG or secoisolariciresinol diglycoside. The SDG is converted by bacteria in the colon to the lignans found in humans and other mammals—enterodiol and enterolactone. These two lignans meet two metabolic fates in our bodies.

1. They can be eliminated directly in food waste (feces) or
2. After being absorbed from the gut, they can travel to the liver and are matched up mainly with glucuronate and excreted in urine or bile. Generally, the more plant lignans you get from your food, the more mammalian lignans you excrete in your urine. So this doesn't sound like lignans are all that important, right? Since they're excreted in urine and all that? Wrong.

DO FLAXSEED LIGNANS HAVE ANTICANCER PROPERTIES?

BASED ON ANIMAL studies, the answer is a resounding "yes." Based on human population studies, the answer is "looks positive." Wouldn't you like to eat something that reduced the size and number of breast tumors in rats? Try flaxseed.

LIGNANS are believed to help protect against hormone-sensitive cancers by inhibiting certain enzymes involved in hormone metabolism, reducing the availability of estrogen, and interfering with tumor cell growth.

FLAX COUNCIL OF CANADA

There have been quite a few very strong rat studies linking flaxseed supplementation (and supplementation with the lignan in flaxseed) with positive changes with breast tissue and tumors. Dr. Lilian Thompson, a recognized researcher in the area of flax and breast cancer, points to studies that suggest flaxseed may lower breast cancer risk in both postmenopausal and premenopausal women.

In one study, rats that already had breast tumors were fed a control diet or the control diet plus the plant lignans or flaxseed. Tumor size was lower in the rats supplementing with the plant lignans and the flax; it is thought that both the lignans and the omega-3s in flaxseed benefit breast tissue. Flaxseed rat studies have also demonstrated a potential protective effect against colon cancer.

After testing the effect of just lignans on human colon tumor cell lines, the researchers concluded that lignans are growth inhibitors of colon tumor cells and they may act through mechanisms other than antiestrogenic activity.

Dr. Wendy Demark-Wahnefried, a diet and prostate researcher at Duke University Medical Center, recently tested the effects of flaxseed-derived lignans on prostate cancer cell lines and found evidence of growth inhibition. The diet was tested out on mice that were genetically programmed to develop prostate cancer and also found the same positive results. This research paper will published in the medical journal *Urology*.

Which brings us to the next obvious question: Do flaxseed and other lignans have anticancer properties in humans? The answer lies somewhere between "perhaps" and "probably." Many human studies are under way, and we'll know more when more results are in. If we look at population studies, they suggest an anticancer role for lignans and other plant estrogens. Basically, researchers have found that populations (such as the Japanese and Chinese) with lower fat, higher fiber diets with high intakes of plant estrogens, including foods rich in lignans have lower incidence of and mortality rates due to breast, endometrial, and prostate cancers.

It is proposed that by interfering with sex hormone metabolism, lignans may protect us against certain cancers, particularly the hormone-sensitive cancers. Lignans have been shown to stimulate synthesis of sex hormone–binding globulin in the liver, which helps to clear out circulating estrogen. Lignans have also been shown to physically bind to estrogen receptors on the sex hormone–binding globulin, which keeps estrogen and testosterone from binding to it. I know this sounds confusing, but here's where it gets interesting.

As these sex hormone–binding globulins, which are bound with lignans instead of estrogen, are found in breast cancer cells, they may be interfering with estrogen-mediated tumorigenic processes taking place there. This is potentially one of the big lignan payoffs.

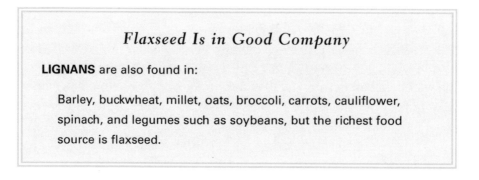

Flaxseed Is in Good Company

LIGNANS are also found in:

Barley, buckwheat, millet, oats, broccoli, carrots, cauliflower, spinach, and legumes such as soybeans, but the richest food source is flaxseed.

Flaxseed has already been shown to reduce breast tumor occurences, and growth of established tumors, in rats. But what about in women? A new study took women that had just been diagnosed with breast cancer and gave half of them a control muffin a day, and half of them a muffin containing 25 grams of flaxseed a day, for thirty-eight days. And guess what happened—the researchers found tumor growth reduced in postmenopausal women who had consumed the flaxseed muffins that compared to the changes they have seen with the drug tamoxifen.

Dr. Lilian Thompson has conducted research on flaxseed for over fifteen years. When Thompson exposed female rats to a carcinogen, after only seven weeks the rats on the flaxseed-supplemented diet had significantly fewer and smaller breast tumors than the group fed a standard diet. Also, male rats fed flaxseed were half as likely to develop colon cancer as those who ate regular rat chow. So, in test-tube and animal studies, it is strongly suspected that flaxseed, probably due to its high phytoestrogen lignan content, may be helpful in shrinking existing breast and colon cancer tumors and stopping new ones from forming. I don't know about you, but this sounds pretty powerful to me.

Lignans are thought to lower cancer risk by blocking some effects of the estrogen your body naturally produces. They are shaped like the human version of estrogen and they may be able to grab on to breast cells, preventing your own estrogen from attaching. Lignans won't stimulate cancerous breast cells to grow, though. Even hot flashes can be lessened for some women with phytoestrogens; a tablespoon of ground flaxseed per day can be very helpful to some women with these symptoms.

Lignans are also thought to boost production of a substance that holds on to human estrogen and carries it out of the body. And if that isn't enough, they are also believed to act as antioxidants, protecting healthy cells from free radicals in the body.

Phytoestrogens in general are linked to decreasing the risk of heart disease and possibly osteoporosis. For example, a recent study concluded that phytoestrogens from soy (soy isoflavones) lessened bone loss from the lumbar spine in perimenopausal women.

Flaxseed Oil Comes Up Short

SINCE most of the lignans are removed from flaxseed during the processing into flaxseed oil, when you use flaxseed oil you are getting the omega-3s in flaxseed but next to none of the fiber and phytoestrogens.

SCIENTIFIC ADVANCEMENTS

The Cancer Connection

Recently, scientists at the National Cancer Institute singled out flaxseed and five other foods as deserving special study because they show potential cancer-fighting abilities. The five other foods are garlic, licorice root, vegetables from the parsnip family, citrus fruits, and soybeans. Preliminary evidence supports the speculation that both the lignans and the plant omega-3 fatty acids in flaxseed may help block substances that promote cancer.

> **BREAST**, prostate, colon, and uterine cancer are the cancers that have been studied in relationship to flaxseed.

The Whole Flax and Nothing but the Flax

We know that flaxseed appears to be protective at the early promotion stage of carcinogenesis, but is it the lignans or the omega-3s in flaxseed that are most helpful? If we take just part of flaxseed (the lignans or the plant omega-3s), will that get the job done? The answer is that we need the whole flax and nothing but the flax. A new study concludes they both help fight cancer, but in different ways and at different times in the carcinogenesis process.

- ❖ The lignans in flaxseed appear to be beneficial throughout the promotional phase of carcinogenisis, whereas the omega-3 component in flax is more effective at the stage when tumors have already been established.
- ❖ Lignans have been proposed to be chemoprotective because they have been shown to inhibit grown of human breast tumor cells, reduce breast tumor initiation, and inhibit the enzyme that boosts the making of estrogen by our bodies.
- ❖ The consumption of flaxseed itself has been found to inhibit breast tumor growth and to reduce early markers of risk for breast and colon carcinogenisis.
- ❖ The omega-3 fatty acids in flaxseed have been shown to reduce breast tumor growth and number in animal studies.
- ❖ Dietary fiber has also been proposed to be chemoprotective because of its influence on sex hormone levels.

Breast Cancer

Thirteen weeks after injecting rats with a breast carcinogen, researchers started supplementing the rats' feed with lignans alone, flaxseed oil alone, or ground flaxseed. After only seven weeks of treatment, the researchers discovered that the size of the breast tumors the rats had before treatment was started were over 50 percent smaller in *all* of the treatment groups. But they also found that the number of new tumors was lowest in the group receiving just the lignans. They concluded that while the lignans in flaxseed appear to be beneficial throughout the promotional phase of carcinogenesis, the oil component of flaxseed (mainly plant omega-3s) is more effective at the stage when tumors have already been established.

From Rats to Women

Estrogen is known to promote tumor growth. Dr. Lilian Thompson explains that flaxseed appears to change the way estrogen is metabolized by the body, making the metabolized product less estrogenic. Another researcher, Dr. Joanne Slavin, lead investigator in a recent flaxseed and breast cancer study, points specifically to the lignan in flaxseed. "Lignan appears to lower estrogen in humans by inhibiting enzymes that are involved in estrogen synthesis," reports Dr. Slavin. In her study, twenty-eight postmenopausal women took daily supplements of 0, 5, or 10 grams of ground flaxseed (10 grams is about 1 tablespoon) in seven-week cycles for a year (their basic diet was about 30 percent calories from fat, 50 percent from carbohydrate, and 20 percent from protein). The 5- and 10-gram groups showed significant decreases in estrogens common to postmenopausal women (estrone sulfate and estradiol). Dr. Slavin suggests that since previous studies show that increased levels of these estrogens may increase a woman's risk of developing breast cancer, reducing levels of these hormones could be protective against breast cancer.

> **"HOPEFULLY** studies will continue to prove they [flaxseeds] have a true protective effect against breast cancer. It would be a wonderful and safe way to gain protection."
>
> —Cindy Moore, M.S., R.D., spokesperson for the American Dietetic Association and Director of Nutrition Therapy of the Cleveland Clinic Foundation

Colon Cancer

Flaxseed has also been shown over the short term to decrease some early markers of colon cancer risk, note two researchers at the University of Toronto in their study article. But in this study they set out to determine whether flaxseed and defatted flaxseed (flaxseed without the plant omega-3s) still exerted a colon cancer–protective effect in rats over a longer period of time. The rats were injected with a colon carcinogen one week before starting the one-hundred-day dietary treatments. While there were cancers and polyps detected in the non-treatment group, the treatment groups were virtually colon cancer–free and had significantly fewer abnormal cavities in their colons as well.

Prostate Cancer

Scientists still cannot say for sure whether flaxseed helps protect against prostate cancer, but so far the evidence looks promising.

The lignans in flaxseed bind testosterone in the gastrointestinal tract and thus may play a role in suppressing the growth of prostate cancer cells, suggests Dr. Demark-Wahnefried. In a pilot study, Dr. Demark-Wahnefried fed twenty-five men, who were waiting to undergo surgery for removal of a cancerous prostate, a thirty-four-day low-fat (20 percent calories from fat), flaxseed-supplemented (30 grams of ground flaxseed per day) diet. She found that on the diet, the men had decreases in serum testosterone (but no decrease in libido or other sexual function), there was a greater rate of tumor cell death while prostate cancer cells were dividing less rapidly, and the levels of PSA (prostate specific antigen—a sign of the presence of prostate cancer) decreased in men with early stage prostate cancer. In the men with more aggressive cancer, the PSA levels continued to rise. Dr. Demark-Wahnefried has already begun a larger study comparing the effects of a low-fat diet with and without flaxseed supplementation on prostate cancer patients.

While Dr. Demark-Wahnefried is not ready to make recommendations for people specifically to consume flaxseed in hopes of cancer prevention, she does agree that as a whole food with a lot of nutrients to its credit, it certainly can be part of a balanced diet.

Research from the University of Virginia Medical School in Charlottesville found a 300 percent increase in the growth of prostate cancer cells with flaxseed oil supplementation. Charles Meyers, M.D., the lead researcher of the study, noted that while there is a negative effect to flax oil, ground flaxseeds might offer some benefit.

Lung Cancer

There's even a study or two on flaxseed and lung cancer. In one recent study, mice that were injected with tumor cells were fed a diet supplemented with lignan isolated from flaxseed two weeks before and after the injection. The lignan-treated group not only had significantly fewer lung tumors, but had smaller tumors as well.

FLAX HELPS THE HEART IN FOUR BIG WAYS

Prepare to be impressed. Flaxseed helps the heart in four ways . . . count them . . . four! The first way you've probably already heard about—**soluble fiber helps reduce cholesterol levels**. Flaxseed has more soluble fiber than oat bran. And we already know that a high intake of soluble fiber may reduce cholesterol levels. Early studies do show that eating flaxseed baked into muffins and breads can lower blood cholesterol levels. Since it is well known that soluble fibers in general, found in fruit pectin and oat bran, for example, are effective cholesterol-lowering food agents, it's likely that the soluble fiber in flaxseed is no exception.

The second way that flax helps the heart is with its **plant omega-3s, which actually do several good things**. Omega-3s suppress the production of a few metabolic bad boys (interleukin-1, tumor necrosis factor, and leukotriene B_4) that are known to encourage the production of oxygen free radicals, which in turn promote the development of hypercholesterolemic atherosclerosis, that is, the accumulation of lipids or plaquing in the arteries.

Flaxseed, after being supplemented in a diet for just one month, may also make our arteries more flexible, helping to maintain a smooth passageway for the blood to pass through, potentially leading to a decreased risk of heart attack and stroke and helping to lower blood pressure.

Atherosclerosis Meets Flaxseed

ATHEROSCLEROSIS is an inflammatory disease. One of the keys to discouraging atherosclerosis is finding interventions that will help alleviate chronic inflammation in the arterial walls. Enter flaxseed.

Flaxseed helps inhibit the production of pro-inflammatory metabolites that occurs from excessive omega-6 fatty acids. This is possibly due to both the plant omega-3s and the lignans in flaxseed.

In one study, researchers measured the effect that consuming two muffins a day (each with 25 grams of flaxseed) for four weeks had on blood lipids in healthy young adults. The levels of omega-3s increased in their plasma lipids and their LDL "bad" cholesterol was reduced by up to 8 percent.

In another study by the same researchers, 50 grams of ground flaxseed eaten with a regular diet for four weeks lowered the LDL cholesterol in healthy adult females by 18 percent.

The third way that flaxseed helps the heart is through its phytoestrogens. **Lignans exhibit anti-inflammatory actions,** meaning they help block the pro-inflammatory actions of platelet activating factor. **Lignans also have antioxidant properties** and may help block the oxidation of LDL "bad" cholesterol particles, encouraging fewer of them to deposit in your arterial walls. The oxidation of LDLs is thought to be a key event in the development of atherosclerosis.

Do You Need Another Reason to Lower Saturated Fat?

BY the way, don't think your strips of bacon are safe yet—substituting plant omega-3s for saturated fat can enhance the beneficial effects of adding flaxseed to your diet, such as the modest reductions in total cholesterol and LDL cholesterol levels.

In one rabbit study, researchers tested the effects of flaxseed on atherosclerosis caused by a high cholesterol diet, the rabbits' lipid levels, and free radical activity. The rabbits were on their treatment diets for eight weeks. The control group, which continued its high-cholesterol ways, had higher total cholesterol values and had marked atherosclerosis in the aorta. The flaxseed-treated rabbits experienced a reduction in the development of aortic atherosclerosis by almost 50 percent. But flaxseed did this without significantly lowering the serum cholesterol.

And now the fourth way: **Omega-3 fatty acids may help prevent cardiac arrhythmias** by enhancing the mechanical performance and electrical stability of the heart. The omega-3s have exhibited antiarrhythmic effects in cell cultures and lab animals and are associated with a reduced risk of fatal ventricular arrhythmia in humans. They may be doing this by modifying the fatty acid composition of cell membrane phospholipids, affecting cell signaling and controlling ion transfers across the cell membrane. Sounds complicated, but the bottom line is—it's a good thing for your heart.

Thin or Round — Flaxseed Doesn't Discriminate

LEAN and obese rats were fed diets containing 20 percent flaxseed meal for six months. The lean rats were hypertensive while the obese rats showed symptoms of type 2 diabetes. The flaxseed decreased total cholesterol and serum triglycerides in both the lean and obese rats.

MY FLAX CHALLENGE
I had my blood lipids and blood pressure taken before I started writing this flax book. Then, for the three months I wrote this book, I ate the way I normally eat and consistently consumed at least 1 tablespoon a day of ground flaxseed (I usually had a tablespoon of ground flax a few times a week). I turned in my book, then literally turned around and tested my blood lipids and blood pressure again. Did it make a difference?

My total cholesterol lowered by 15mg/dl and my LDL cholesterol went down by 5.

FLAX MAY REDUCE BLOOD CLOTS AND STROKE

THE OMEGA-3 fatty acids in flaxseed help prevent blood clots that might lead to heart attacks, according to University of Toronto researcher Stephen Cunnane, Ph.D. The omega-3s do this by helping make platelets or less likely to stick together, thus avoiding a chain reaction that leads to a blood clot. How incredible is that? For this reason alone, every American should be finding ways to eat flax.

Feel the Power

ONE study, which found that as the plant omega-3 content of blood cholesterol esters and phospholipids went up, the risk of stroke went down, calculated that each standard deviation increase in plant omega-3s (ALA) was associated with a 30 percent reduction in stroke risk.

One study showed that taking in some omega-3 fatty acids once a heart attack took place decreased the rate of cardiac death—due to the antiarrhythmic properties of omega-3s. Fish oil, a particularly potent source of omega-3s, has been shown to reduce ventricular arrhythmias and to be more beneficial than various pharmacologic agents on the market.

FLAX MAY DELAY THE DEVELOPMENT OF TYPE 2 DIABETES

TYPE 2 DIABETES has reached epidemic proportions in this country and I've got to admit, I'm always a bit nervous every time I give my urine sample during a physical exam. My father had type 2 diabetes and I've written two books on diet and type 2 diabetes, and suffice it to say—I don't want it. I never expected to find anything remotely related to type 2 diabetes when I started my literature review on flaxseed. But, lo and behold, flaxseed was recently shown to delay type 2 diabetes in rats. I'm jumping up and down over this news.

The antioxidant-acting lignan found in flaxseed, secoisolariciresinol diglucoside (SDG), was isolated from flaxseed and given via the drinking water to a type of female rat (Zucker diabetic fatty rats) that is susceptible to a rodent analog of human type 2 diabetes. By day seventy-two, 100 percent of the control rats not receiving lignans from flaxseed had developed type 2 diabetes as compared to 20 percent of the lignan-treated rats. By day 101, all but 10 percent of the treated rats had developed diabetes.

> The soluble fiber in flaxseed may also benefit people with diabetes by reducing their blood glucose response to carbohydrates. This would help normalize blood sugars and might help discourage obesity as well.

FLAX HELPS REGULATE THE BOWELS AND PREVENT CONSTIPATION

GROUND FLAXSEED INCREASES stool weight and improves laxation. There—I said it. It isn't pretty, but it sure comes in handy when you are trying to stay regular.

The fact that flaxseed contains both soluble and insoluble fiber makes it particularly helpful in keeping our intestines happy. The insoluble fiber in flax, like the fiber in wheat bran, adds bulk as the food waste moves through the intestines, while the soluble fiber blends with water in the intestines and forms a gel-like mixture that gently helps soften the stool, moving it through the colon more quickly.

One study of healthy young adults found that when they ate 50 grams of flaxseed a day (by eating two 25-gram flaxseed muffins), their bowel movements per week increased by 30 percent.

But what if increasing bowel movements is the last thing you need? Personally, I have diarrhea-predominant IBS (Irritable Bowel Syndrome), which basically means that I battle frequent, urgent stools. Suffice it to say, constipation is not a word in my vocabulary. While I was writing this book, I had 1 to 2 tablespoons of ground flaxseed every day and I must say, I think this regular dose of flax actually helped my IBS. It definitely didn't hurt it, but of course not everyone's IBS is the same and your intestines may react differently.

FLAXSEED DELIVERS A ONE-TWO PUNCH
TO BOOST YOUR IMMUNE SYSTEM

FLAXSEED BOOSTS YOUR immune system in two ways. The first punch comes from the plant omega-3s, followed by a quick hit from the lignans. Research suggests that they both moderate the immune response and may play a beneficial role in the clinical management of "hyper-stimulated" immune and inflammatory diseases such as rheumatoid arthritis, psoriasis and eczema, multiple sclerosis, systematic lupus erythmatosis, and ulcerative colitis.

- ❖ **Punch One**—plant omega-3s work by suppressing lymphocyte proliferation and cytokine production and by changing the fatty acid makeup of membrane phospholipids, which ultimately decrease the production of pro-inflammatory substances (eicosanoids, leukotriene B_4 [LTB_4] and thromboxane A_2 [TXA_2]), while enhancing the production of less inflammatory substances (prostaglandin I_3 [PGI_3], and the less damaging eicosanoids).
- ❖ **Punch Two**—Lignans work by favorably influencing certain mediators of the immune response. Lignans are potent inhibitors of platelet-activating factor (a mediator of inflammation). A recent study seems to indicate that lignans can help improve renal function in lupus nephritis patients. The patients consumed 15 to 45 grams of flaxseed per day for four weeks.

FLAX MAY HELP RELIEVE SYMPTOMS OF RHEUMATOID ARTHRITIS

THE OMEGA-3 fatty acids found in flaxseed seem to have an anti-inflammatory effect on patients with rheumatoid arthritis, reducing morning stiffness and joint tenderness.

There is consistent evidence from well-designed studies (double blind, placebo-controlled clinical trials) that omega-3 fatty acids supplied as fish oil can have modest beneficial effects in rheumatoid arthritis. It is suggested that these modest effects could become more powerful with a lower omega-6 fatty acid diet, as omega-6s compete with omega-3s in the body and too much omega-6 in the diet makes it more difficult for omega-3s to do their job. It is possible that the omega-3s in flaxseed, along with a reduction in omega-6s in your daily diet, could help contribute to this beneficial anti-inflammatory effect from fish omega-3s. Researchers suspect that omega-3s help suppress the production of inflammatory mediators such as the omega-6 eicosanoids and pro-inflammatory cytokines.

The bottom line is that making smarter diet choices can complement the drugs people with rheumatoid arthritis are already taking. Increasing omega-3s and decreasing omega-6s can possibly have drug-sparing effects.

Flax May Help Relieve Breast Pain Related to a Woman's Hormone Cycle

Not only can breast pain be extremely uncomfortable, it also has sometimes been associated with breast cancer risk. Flaxseed is an attractive, low-cost, low-risk alternative for controlling symptoms, an alternative to hormonal therapy, which can come with side effects and potential risks with long-term use. Researchers at the University of Toronto recently tested the effect that a daily dose of flaxseed might have for women with breast pain. Over a six-month period, fifty-six premenopausal women ate a 25-gram flaxseed-containing muffin per day and sixty premenopausal women ate a placebo muffin. The women eating the flaxseed-containing muffin experienced significantly greater breast pain reduction than the control group—possibly due to an anti-estrogenic effect of the lignans in flaxseed. And the best part was that all this relief took place with no significant side effects observed by the flaxseed therapy group.

Why Is It So Important to Grind the Flaxseed?

Once you grind the flaxseeds—and you'll want to, because the body enzymes get to the beneficial chemical components better this way—it is highly perishable; it lasts only a week in the refrigerator. So I recommend grinding a month's worth of flaxseed at a time—I use an electric coffee grinder—and keeping it in a Ziploc bag or an opaque airtight container in the freezer. This way it will be as fresh as possible and will keep in the freezer for a month or more. You can eat it straight from the freezer, too—there's no need to defrost.

FLAXSEED + FISH = BIG BENEFITS

I KNOW WHAT you are thinking, but just because you are going to be supplementing with flax almost every day doesn't mean you should stop eating fish a couple of times a week. The omegas that we get from fish benefit our bodies in different ways than the omegas we get from flaxseed. We need them both.

A researcher from the Lyon Diet Study, whose participants had previously survived a heart attack, found that it was the plant omega-3 (ALA) and not the fish omega-3s (EPA and DHA) that was significantly associated with protection against recurrence of heart attacks. Other studies have also suggested that the cardiovascular effects of the plant omega-3 are different from those of fish.

When you eat lots of wonderful plant omega-3s, it leads to a significant increase of the long-chain omega-3 (EPA) in body tissue levels, but not so much of the other long chain omega-3 found in fish (DHA). But when we eat fish—which contains both EPA and DHA—we see higher concentrations of both EPA and DHA in our body tissues.

2

Flaxseed 101

101 Important Tips and Facts about Flax—How to Buy It, Grind It, Store It, Add It, and Much More

So, you want to add flaxseed to your daily diet. You've read about how amazing it is for your health. Maybe there's even a bag of ground flaxseed that you bought a month ago, sitting in your refrigerator as we speak. And each time you open the refrigerator door, you look at it and wonder what you're going to do with it.

Wonder no more. The following 101 quick tips offer you some real-life flaxseed advice and options, so each person can customize her own plan for adding flaxseed into her busy day.

Once you get past the flaxseed basics—how to buy it, grind it, and store it—you will want and need to know what to do with this powerful plant. Stirring it into your orange juice or hot oatmeal gets pretty old by the third or fourth week. Trust me.

Over the last couple of years, scores of people who have heard about the benefits of flaxseed have written in (via my website www.recipedoctor.com), asking "Do you have recipes that will help me get my daily dose of flaxseed?" Well, folks, that's what *The Flax Cookbook* is all about—answering that one crucial question. Up until now, for most health-minded people, flaxseed has been on the fringe of American society, making its way (if it gets lucky) into an occasional smoothie or bowl of oatmeal. With this book we are going to crank it up a few notches. I want to take flaxseed to a place it's never been before, front and center in our minds, in our kitchens, and most importantly, in our daily diet.

Below you will find literally over one hundred facts about flax, starting with general flax facts, then moving into tips on buying, grinding, storing, and adding flax to your diet. I hope that by the time you've finished this chapter, you'll feel very "Zen" about flax—like you know everything there is to know about the care and uses of flax.

FLAX HISTORY

1. The Babylonians cultivated flaxseed as early as 3,000 B.C.
2. In 650 B.C., Hippocrates used flax for the relief of intestinal discomfort.
3. In the eighth century, King Charlemagne passed laws and regulations governing flaxseed consumption.

GENERAL FLAX FACTS

4. **Flaxseed tops many nutrition charts**
    Flaxseed is the richest food source of the plant omega-3 fatty acid, linolenic acid, and lignans on the planet.
5. **Good things come in small packages**
    Flax is a tiny, oval, reddish-brown seed (it looks a little like a sesame seed) that has a pleasant, nutty taste. When ground up (not too fine) it can take you back to the '70s—it looks not unlike wheat germ. When golden flax (a lighter-colored type of flaxseed) is ground up fairly finely, it looks a little like cornmeal.
6. **Flaxseed boasts both types of fiber**
    Flaxseed contains both soluble and insoluble fiber. Each level tablespoon of ground flax contains about 2½ to 3 grams of fiber. The fiber may be a little more or less depending on the brand.

7. **Some say golden flax is where it's at**

    Golden flax is another type of flaxseed that has a lighter, golden color. Some marketers of golden flax may claim that it has even more of the good stuff than the regular, brownish flaxseed. But data compiled by the Canadian Grain Commission showed that as flaxseed production moves south, the flax crop tends to produce seeds with higher protein, less oil, and a lower omega-3 content, and golden flax tends to be grown further south in North and South Dakota. Golden flax is usually more expensive than the darker flaxseed.

8. **Golden is easier on the eyes**

    The one advantage I can see to golden flax is that the lighter color makes it a little easier to hide in dishes and recipes. For testing the recipes in this book, though, I used regular flax most of the time. I figured if I could develop tips and recipes to help you all consume (and sometimes hide) the darker flaxseed, well, then, I was only going to be ahead of the golden flax game. I did specify in some recipes to use golden flaxseed when the lighter color flax would truly work best due to its color.

9. **More brown flax is grown commercially than golden flax and it's therefore easier to find in stores.**

    I live in California and had to go to a certain health food store to get golden flax. But golden is available for purchase on several flaxseed websites, including the obvious www.goldenflax.com.

10. **All flax brands are not created equal**

    It would be incorrect for me to say that one tablespoon of ground flaxseed contains 30 calories, 2 grams of fiber, and 2 grams of omega-3 fatty acid because all of this depends on the particular brand and grind of the flax. One tablespoon of Bob's Red Mill Flaxseed Meal (packaged ground flaxseed) weighs in at 6.5 grams and contains:

    30 calories
    2.25 grams of total fat
    2 grams carbohydrate
    2 grams of fiber
    1.5 grams protein

But 1 tablespoon of another brand of ground flaxseed, Ultra Omega Balance, weighs in at 15 grams and contains:

75 calories

5 grams of total fat

5 grams carbohydrate

4 grams fiber

3 grams protein

See my problem? I looked in my nutrition database and found a flaxseed code that seemed to fall somewhere in the middle. That's what I used to analyze the recipes and that's what I used below.

11. **If flax had a nutrition label**

Flaxseed

Serving Size: 1 tablespoon ground flaxseed (8.13 grams)

Calories = 40

Protein = 1.6 g

Carbohydrate = 2.8 g

Total Fat = 2.7 g

Saturated Fat = 0.26 g

Monounsaturated Fat = 0.6 g

Polyunsaturated Fat = 1.8 g

Cholesterol = 0 mg

Total Fiber = 2.3 g

Sodium = 3 mg

Omega-3 fatty acids = 1.5 g

Omega-6 fatty acids = 0.3 g

Vitamins and minerals

Vitamin B_6 = 6% RDA

Vitamin E = 6% DV

Folic Acid = 15% DV

Iron = 4% DV

Magnesium = 12.5% DV

Phosphorus = 6% DV

12. **Don't be shocked by the fat grams**

Flaxseed is about 40 percent oil, more than half of which is a plant form of an omega-3 fatty acid. So when you add flaxseed to your recipes, realize that the grams of fat are going to increase per serving. Granted, they are fat grams well spent, but it does take some getting used to. As a nutrition author and national columnist who is used to taking out extra fat and calories from recipes, I'm rather used to watching the calories and fat grams go down in my recipes. But the good news is, the fat and calories are going to go up only a little. If you add a tablespoon of ground flaxseed per serving, the calories and fat grams will bump up about 30 calories and 2.2 grams of fat per serving.

13. **More omega-3s than canola and soybeans**

Since flaxseed is 40 percent oil and contains an impressive amount of plant omega-3s, it isn't surprising that flaxseed "oil" actually contains more plant omega-3s than two other oils known for containing omega-3s—canola and soybean oil.

14. **It's two fibers in one!**

Flaxseed is actually a good source of both types of fiber, soluble and insoluble. We talk more about the soluble fiber in flaxseed in this book because that's the fiber that's associated with blood sugar and cholesterol lowering benefits. And that's the type of fiber that is harder to get in grains and other plant foods. Having soluble fiber is what gave oat bran its day in the sun.

How to Buy Flax

15. **A buck a pound!**

Flaxseed is sold as whole, unground seeds for around $.99 a pound in the bulk food section of your local health food store. That's the deal of the century if you ask me. This is the price for the regular type of flaxseed with the darker brown seed color. You will have to grind it yourself, but the price is still right.

16. **How far will a pound of flax go?**

A pound of whole flaxseed will transform into about 68 tablespoons of ground flaxseed (4¼ cups). If you make a point to add a tablespoon of ground flaxseed a day to your diet, a pound of whole flaxseed will buy you about a two-month supply of ground flaxseed for one person, or a one-month supply for a couple.

17. **Do the math**

If a pound of flax gives you about a two-month supply of ground flaxseed (one tablespoon a day) and a pound of whole flax costs around a dollar a pound, you are paying about fifty cents a month—which computes to less than two cents a day—to give yourself one of the most powerful plant foods on the planet. You can't even get a stick of gum for that price.

18. **Upscale flaxseed**

If you are buying golden flax, you will have to dig a little deeper into that pocket. A pound of golden flax will run you about $1.60 a pound (still a good deal, in my book) if you buy it in bulk at a local health food store.

19. **Now for something completely convenient**

Packages of "flax meal" are available at some health food and grocery stores in one-pound bags for about three dollars. Flax meal is basically ground flaxseed. Nothing more, nothing less. It's still a good idea to keep your bag of flax meal in the freezer—preventing it from becoming rancid and keeping the flavors fresh—and just spoon it out when you need it.

20. **A flax by any other name**

Although the terms *flax* and *flaxseed* are by far the most common names for flaxseed, it is also known as:

Linum usitatissimum
Linseed-Lint bells
Linum
winterlien

21. **Where to buy your flax**

These are your options, depending on where you live. You can buy whole flaxseed or flaxmeal (both packaged in 1 pound bags) at some of your local grocery stores. You can go to your closest health food store and buy it in bulk by the pound and grind it at home. Or you can order it whole or ground over the Internet.

22. **Surfing the Net for flax**

There are lots of companies selling flaxseed over the Internet but these are the ones I found easily when I did my own Internet search:

www.bobsredmill.com (1 pound bag of golden flax for $2.16)
www.goldenflax.com (4½ pounds of milled golden flax for $22,
    12 pounds of whole golden flax for $38)

www.oldtimeherbs.com (1 pound bag of whole flaxseed for $2.95,
    1 pound bag of organic flax meal for $4.50)
www.flaxproducts.com (1 pound milled flax in plastic jars for $8.99)
The flax council website also has a list of flaxseed suppliers. You can
    visit the flax council at www.flaxcouncil.ca

BACK TO THE GRIND

23. **Get into the grind**

    Grinding flaxseeds breaks them up, making them easier to digest and the nutrients more available to the body. You've got to grind the flaxseed to make all the lignans, omega-3s, and soluble fiber available to your body's digestive system.

24. **You're supplementing your sewer**

    If you just sprinkle whole flaxseeds over your cereal or in your breads or casseroles, you are just supplementing your sewer because the whole flaxseed passes right through your system, still intact. Which means most of the nutrients inside the flaxseed aren't getting absorbed into your body.

25. **From wheat germ to cornmeal consistency**

    You can use a coffee grinder, food processor, or blender to grind flaxseed. If you grind them briefly you will get a coarse, flaky grind, similar to wheat germ. If you process longer and harder, you will get a finer ground flaxseed, similar to the consistency of cornmeal. (I prefer the finer grind.)

26. **Got coffee grinders?**

    One of the best ways I've found to grind flaxseed is using one of those 6-inch, zippy little electric coffee grinders. I've got a Krups brand coffee grinder in my kitchen. My husband buys his coffee beans whole so we actually use it for both purposes. He goes on record as saying that he hates that I use "his" coffee grinder for "my" flaxseed. So, while he is safely at work, I just grind a month's worth of flaxseed all at once, then I carefully clean the coffee grinder out, removing any evidence of flaxseed. My flaxseed does seem to have a slight essence of coffee flavoring, but I love the flavor of coffee, so that's a good thing.

27. **Have "his" and "hers" coffee grinders**

   If you don't want to battle a spouse or roommate over the coffee grinder, just have "his" and "hers" coffee grinders. Buy a second one and write the words "flaxseed only" on it with a permanent marker, or place a sticker to that effect on the front of it. The average electric coffee grinder can be yours for about twenty-five dollars.

28. **A grinder made just for flaxseed**

   There's a company out in Internet Land that is selling a grinder specifically for flaxseed. It looks a lot like those little electric coffee grinders and it's priced a lot like them, too ($29). You can check it out at www.ageless.com/flaxseed.htm.

HOW TO STORE FLAX

29. **You've got a year**

   Whole flax (unground), as long as it is dry and of good quality, can be stored at room temperature for up to a year. So, if you're like me, and you tend to trek over to your local health food store about every six months, just buy a six-month supply of whole flaxseed and keep it in the back of your dark and dry kitchen cabinet, grinding it as needed.

30. **No need for sunscreen**

   It's best to shield flaxseed (ground or whole) from light. So, once it is ground, just store flaxseed in an opaque container in the refrigerator, or better yet, the freezer. Store flax as directed on the package if you are using commercially ground flaxseed; you'll notice flax meal companies tend to use dark brown packaging.

31. **Flaxseed enthusiasts, contain yourself**

   The minute you grind those flaxseeds, all those wonderful unsaturated fatty acids become more vulnerable to mixing with oxygen and other items from the air. So, pour your just-ground flaxseed into an airtight (as well as opaque) bag or container and put it immediately into the refrigerator or freezer. It will keep well there for up to two months.

32. **A place in the sun . . . NOT!**

   The omega-3 fatty acids in flax are susceptible to oxidation because these fatty acids have three double bonds in their carbon chain, and double bonds are just itching to mix it up with oxygen. Warm temperatures and light both encourage the oxidation process in general. This gives us the best reason to keep our ground flaxseed in the freezer.

33. **The omega-3 fatty acids in whole flax are remarkably resistant to oxidation, according to lab tests.**

    The outside of the flaxseed appears to keep the fatty acids well protected. I still think it's a good idea to keep your whole flax in a dark, cool kitchen cabinet, though.

How to Add Flax

34. **Got water?**

    If you are increasing the fiber in your diet—and supplementing with flax—you should always be sure to drink plenty of water. Lots of fiber or flax, with too little fluid, can lead to a blockage in the intestines.

35. **Stick to the seeds, not pills or potions**

    It isn't advised to take different formulations of flax at the same time (tablets, liquids, etc.) Overdosing on flax is more likely this way. Stick to the most natural form of flax—the ground flaxseed. It's got all the nutrients you need from flax. It's usually best to turn to the most natural form of a food instead of a pill or potion.

36. **Less flour, more flax**

    Since ground flaxseed's texture is similar to that of wheat bran, bakers tend to substitute ground flaxseed for a small amount of the flour in baked goods. Ground flax is mostly made up of fiber, protein, and fatty acids and it looks and acts more like a grain than anything else. So, if you are trying to add it to your bakery recipes, try replacing ¼ to ½ cup of the flour with ground flaxseed if the recipe calls for two or more cups of flour. This will work in your muffin, bread, and biscuit recipes.

37. **More is not better in baked recipes**

    Adding too much flaxseed to a recipe can result in lower volume baked goods, which means they won't rise as high or be as airy. Commercial bakers often add extra gluten to help compensate for this.

38. **Flax instead of oil?**

    One reference I read suggested substituting flax for the oil called for in a recipe. For example, they suggested adding a cup of flax instead of ⅓ cup oil. I can't personally see this working. While oil is a liquid that adds liquid volume and moisture to a recipe, flax is a high-oil seed that, when ground, is flaky—similar in texture to a whole grain. See my point?

39. **Top it with flaxseed, too**

    You can also sprinkle some ground flax on top of each muffin, roll, or bread loaf before baking. You can even make a topping mixture of oats and ground flaxseed if you'd like. To add a little glisten, spray the tops with a bit of canola cooking spray before and after.

40. **Look for low-fat recipes**

    Since ground flaxseed contains a hefty dose of fatty acids (mostly omega-3 fatty acids—so this is good), it works best to add ground flax to lower-fat recipes. This way you won't be adding more fatty acids to a recipe already maxed out on grams of fat.

NON-COOKS WHO STILL WANT TO ADD FLAX

41. **Have you had your flax sprinkle today?**

    If you are the type of person that just wants to wash down the flaxseed dose and be done with it, you can always stir a tablespoon of ground flaxseed into ½ cup of orange juice or similar liquid and just drink it down.

42. **Fruit is your flaxseed friend**

    Sprinkle a tablespoon of ground flaxseed or a scoop of flaxseed containing cereal (¼ cup or more) over berries, sliced peaches, or any fresh fruit you enjoy.

43. **Yodel for yogurt**

    One of my favorite quick-and-easy ways to add flax is just to stir a tablespoon into my container of yogurt. I like the four-ounce containers of Dannon La Crème yogurt, but you can add it to whatever yogurt you like, even key lime or cappuccino-flavored yogurt. You literally just peel off the top, measure a tablespoon of your ground flaxseed, and pour it in. Carefully stir it all together right there in the container, and you are good to go!

44. **Make a flaxseed yogurt parfait**

Make a flaxseed yogurt parfait by topping a serving of your favorite yogurt with some fresh fruit and then topping that with some grand flaxseed-containing granola (see table of cereals containing flaxseed on page 48). It's so delicious you won't even notice it's good for you.

45. **Take your lumps**

Stir a tablespoon of ground flax and some fruit into your serving of cottage cheese for a quick snack.

46. **B.Y.O.F.**

Bring Your Own (ground) Flaxseed with you in a Ziploc plastic bag or tiny Tupperware-like container, so you can stir it into the smoothies or iced coffee drinks you buy at those convenient smoothie or coffee chain stores.

47. **Supplement your soy drink with flax**

Stir a tablespoon or two of ground flaxseed into a favorite soy drink. Some soymilk brands taste better than others do, so the key is to find one that you like.

48. **Make your own hot or cold flaxseed cereal**

You don't have to buy hot or cold flaxseed-containing cereals—you can make a quick batch at home. Prepare your hot or cold cereal the way you like it, then sprinkle a teaspoon or tablespoon of ground flax over the top and stir.

49. **Sandwich flax into your lunch**

Sprinkle a teaspoon or two of ground flaxseed onto the spicy mustard, chutney, cheese spread, or peanut butter you use to dress your sandwich.

50. to 80. **It's already in there**

Buy these products and you'll get a dose of ground flaxseed. How easy is that? The following food products contain ground flaxseed as an ingredient, which is really convenient because it saves you the work of grinding it yourself. Below, you'll see where you can go to get them, whether you can buy them over the Internet, and even how much ground flaxseed is in a serving of each product (if that information is available). The reason I didn't include products that contain whole flaxseed is because the nutrients in whole (unground) flaxseed are mostly unavailable to the body.

Food Products in Canada/USA
Containing Ground Flaxseed

Breads	*Product Name*	*Where You Can Find It*
Dimpflmeier Bakery Ltd. (Beckmann & Markner Inc.) P.O. Box 207 Grimsby, ON Canada L3M 4G3	•Linseed/flax (Leinsamen) •100% Rye with Linseed •7 Grain	Order by phone or Internet 800-723-8823 www.dimpfbreadex.com
Oroweat Bread (Bimbo Bakeries U.S.A.) Montebello, CA U.S.A.	•Buttermilk 9 Grain •Best Winter Wheat Premier •Old Country 10 Grain	Available in supermarkets across the U.S. and parts of Canada.

Cereals

Bob's Red Mill Natural Foods, 5209 Southeast International Way Milwauki, OR 97222 U.S.A. 503-654-3215	•5 Grain Rolled Hot Cereal (contains rolled oats, wheat, rye, barley, triticale, and flaxseed) •7 Grain Cereal •Apple Cinnamon Grains •10 Grain Hot Cerea (contains milled wheat, rye triticale, oats, oat bran, corn, barley, soy beans, brown rice, millet, and flaxseed)	Available across the U.S.A. and parts of Canada. Use the "storefinder" on the Web site to find store locations: www.bobsredmill.com

Taster's Note: The 5 Grain Rolled Cereal can be used in recipes instead of regular rolled oats.

Food By Design, Inc. 1850 Blucher Valley Rd. P.O. Box 1474 Sebastopol, CA U.S.A. 415-563-1661	•Healthy Scoop (contains golden flax, organic oats, soy flour, brown rice, and maple syrup)	Available in natural foods stores across Northern California and can be ordered on the Web site: www.foodbydesign.com

Taster's note: This cereal tastes great mixed with yogurt and fruit, and has 2.8 grams omega-3s per ½-cup serving.

Nature's Path Foods 7453 Progress Way Delta, BC Canada V4G1E8 888-808-9505	•Nature's Path Flax Plus[1] •Nature's Path Mesa •Sunrise Flakes[2] •Nature's Path Optimum	Available in natural food stores across North America and in some major grocery stores, as well as

Cereals	*Product Name*	*Where You Can Find It*
	•Power Breakfast[3]	on the Web site: www.naturespath.com

[1]Flax Plus contains 1.8-2.0 grams of flaxseed per 30 gram serving.
[2]Mesa Sunrise contains 2.2-2.5 grams of flaxseed per 30 gram serving.
[3]Optimum Power contains 2.7-2.9 grams of flaxseed per 55 grams serving.
(All three of these cereals contain partially ground flaxseed.)

Robin Hood Multifoods Inc 60 Columbia Way Markham, ON Canada L3R OC9 800-268-3232	•Ready to Serve Red River Cereal •Original Red River Cereal •Maple & Brown Sugar	Available in stores only in Canada, but available in the U.S.A. through Mille Lacs Corp. (800-626-3809) www.redrivercereal.com

The Red River cereal contains ground and whole flaxseed—adding up to a total of 5 grams of flaxseed per serving.

Health Valley Company (Hanes Celestial Co.) 1600 Foothill Blvd. Irwindale, CA 91706 800-423-4846	•Organic Golden Flax cereal	Available for purchase at health food stores across the U.S.A. and in the Naturemart Web site: www.naturemart.com

Prairie Sun Grains 2000 Inc. Box 1570 Camrose, AB Canada T4V 1X4 780-672-3675	•Prairie Sun Certified Flax •Organic Hot Cereal	Available in supermarkets across western Canada and in some stores in eastern Canada.

Zoe Foods
49 Winchester St.
Newton, MA 02461
877-415-3663
	Varieties include:
	•Zoe Flax & Soy Granola:
	  cranberries and currants
	  almonds and oats
	  apple cinnamon
	  (each contains ground
	  flaxseed, roasted soy-
	  beans, crisped soy
	  nuggets, isolated soy
	  protein, rolled oats, honey, etc.
		Available in 1,100 stores
		across U.S.A. (natural
		foods stores and super-
		markets such as Whole
		Foods). Use the "store-
		finder" on Web site to find
		store locations:
		www.zoefoods.com

Each ⅔-cup serving of cereal contains 1 tablespoon of ground flax, adding about 2.4 grams omega 3s.

Cereals	_Product Name_	_Where You Can Find It_

Taster's note: I love the apple cinnamon granola. It has lots of flavor and is very moist for a granola. It works well stirred into yogurt or topping a bowl of fresh fruit.

Energy Bars

Zoe Foods
49 Winchester St.
Newton, MA 02461
877-415-3663

•Zoe Flax & Soy Bars
4 flavors:
chocolate
peanut butter
apple crisp
lemon

Available in 1,100 stores across U.S.A. (natural food supermarkets such as Whole Foods). Use the "storefinder" on the Web site to find store locations: www.zoefoods.com

Each bar contains 1 tablespoon of ground flaxseed.

Taster's note: These bars are moist and have a nice flavor. My favorite flavor is the lemon, but my children like the chocolate and peanut butter flavors better.

Food By Design, Inc.
1850 Blucher Valley Rd.
P.O. Box 1474
Sebastopol, CA U.S.A.
415-563-1661

•Healthy Break Bar
(contains soy, flax, organic oats, brown rice syrup, honey, cinnamon, etc.)

Available in natural foods stores across northern California and can be ordered on the Web site: www.foodbydesign.com

Each bar contains 1.7 grams of omega-3s.

Taster's note: This bar is lightly sweet and nicely moist and chewy.

Mixes

Pizzey's Milling
Box 132
Angusville, Manitoba
Canada R0J 0A0
800-804-6433

•Flax 'n Bran Muffin Mix
(contains whole wheat flour, brown sugar, whey powder, milled flaxseed, organic unbleached flour, dehydrated molasses, salt, baking powder, and cinnamon)
•Flax Pancake & Waffle Mix
(contains whole wheat flour, unbleached white flour, milled flaxseed, baking powder, salt)

Available through their 800 number (at left) and their Web site: www.pizzeys.com

If desired you can use ¼ cup egg substitute in place of the egg called for in these mixes' directions and use canola oil when oil is called for.

Mixes	_Product Name_	_Where You Can Find It_
Bob's Red Mill Natural Foods 5209 Southeast International Way Milwauki, OR 97222 U.S.A. 503-654-3215	•10 Grain Pancake & Waffle Mix	Available across the U.S.A. and parts of Canada. Use the "storefinder" on the Web site to find store locations: www.bobsredmill.com
Nunweiler's Flour Co. 106-129 Commercial Way Penicton, BC Canada V2A 3H4 888-726-2253 (888-PANCAKE)	•Wheat n' Flax Pancake and Waffle Mix	Available through the Web site: www.pancakemix.com

Any type of milk can be used in this mix, even soy or rice milk, and egg substitute can also be used.

FLAXSEED WARNINGS

81. **The FDA is not on the case . . . yet**
    Flax has not yet been evaluated by the Food and Drug Administration for safety, effectiveness, or purity.

82. The U.S. has not released a recommended intake of omega fatty acids (3s or 6s). But remember—flaxseed is a wonderful source of plant omega-3s.

83. **If allergic, beware**
    It's rare, but a small number of people do have allergic reactions to flax. Stop taking flax and seek emergency medical attention immediately if you experience any of the following symptoms:
    ❖ difficulty breathing
    ❖ the feeling that your throat is closing
    ❖ swelling of your lips, tongue, or face
    ❖ hives

84. **Talk to your doctor first**
    Do not try flax without first talking with your doctor if you have a medical condition, specifically:
    ❖ narrowing of the esophagus or another stomach area
    ❖ intestinal obstruction or other stomach or intestinal problems

❖ prostate problems

❖ difficulty with urination

85. **Ask first, if there is a bun is in the oven**

Do not take flax without first talking to your doctor if you are pregnant or could become pregnant. It is not yet known with certainty that flax will not harm an unborn baby.

86. **Same goes for breastfeeding**

Do not take flax without first talking to your doctor if you are breastfeeding your baby. It is not yet known with certainty that flax will not harm a nursing infant. Some of the phytoestrogens and omega-3 fatty acids in the flaxseed you eat might get into the breastmilk and be passed on to your nursing baby.

87. **Flax gets a PG rating**

There is no information available yet on whether children can consume flaxseed on a frequent or occasional basis. You should always consult your child's doctor before giving them any herbal/health supplement and flaxseed is no exception.

88. **Any allergies to plants?**

If you have allergies, especially to plants, talk to your doctor or pharmacist before starting a flaxseed regimen.

89. **What else are you taking?**

Consult with your doctor or pharmacist before you start supplementing your diet with flax if you are taking other medicines or other herbal/health supplements—flaxseed might decrease the absorption of some drugs when taken together. Therefore, flax may not be recommended in some situations. Find out for sure first. Medical professionals may advise you to consume flaxseed a certain number of hours before or after you take your medication.

90. **Is that a balloon in your stomach?**

Because of the higher soluble fiber content of flax, it binds with water (causing it to swell) and forms a gel-like mixture. This is why it may be dangerous if used by people with certain intestinal problems. If you keep your flaxseed dose down to one tablespoon at a time, you will most likely be minimizing this swelling effect.

91. **How irritable is your bowel?**

I have Irritable Bowel Syndrome (the diarrhea-predominant type) and never noticed any problems with flaxseed exacerbating my symptoms. I did, however, make a point never to have more than two tablespoons of ground flax per day. I don't know if it was wishful thinking, but shortly after being more faithful about having flaxseed at least once a day, I did notice that my morning symptoms seemed to improve. Everybody's irritable bowels are different though, so keep that in mind as you try out some of these tips.

92. **Too much of a good thing?**

At the time of publication, no symptoms of flax overdose were known, other than the previously mentioned warnings of the potential for intestinal blockages in susceptible people.

Bake It . . . Bake It Good

93. **Flax is gluten-free**

You don't want to substitute too much flax for the flour in recipes because flax doesn't have the gluten (vegetable protein) that flour does. And breads need gluten to create gluten strands, which help give bread its airy structure. You can get away with substituting some of the flour though, say, ¼ cup ground flaxseed with every two cups of flour, or a ratio of about 1 to 8.

94. **Baking doesn't bake off the plant omega-3s**

The omega-3s in whole and milled (ground) flaxseed appear to be stable to the baking temperatures typical of breads and muffins. According to the Flax Council of Canada, studies have shown the omega-3 content of milled flax virtually unchanged after baking at 350°F for two hours.

95. **Boiling doesn't bother the plant omega-3s**

North Dakota State University studied the effect of processing and cooking on the stability of alpha-linolenic acid (the omega-3 in flaxseed) in spaghetti fortified with ground flaxseed. The researchers found that the plant omegas remained stable.

96. **Lignans are safe to heat, too**

According to the Flax Council of Canada, several studies suggest there is no significant loss of the lignans (phytoestrogens) from flax during the baking process.

97. **Raw versus baked**

A group of nine young women included 50 grams of flax in their daily diet for a month. Half of them added ground flaxseed to breakfast cereals, soup, juice, or yogurt. The other half ate bread baked with ground flax rather than their usual bread. Plasma fatty acid values during the month did not differ significantly between the two groups. Incidentally, both groups lowered their serum total cholesterol and their LDL "bad" cholesterol.

98. **It browns while it bakes**

Because baked foods made with flaxseed brown rapidly, watch cooking times carefully when you are changing a bakery recipe to include some flaxseed.

99. **How (and where) does your flaxseed grow?**

Where your flaxseed is grown does determine how much lignan is in your tablespoon of flaxseed. Researchers at the University of Toronto found significant differences in lignan content of different varieties of flaxseed, ranging from .96 mumol/gram for the Linott variety to 3.15 mumol/gram for the Somme variety of flaxseed. Growing location had significant effects on the lignan content from all the varieties of flax.

POTENTIAL NEGATIVE EFFECTS OF ADDING FIBER TO YOUR DIET

100. **Calories can pass right through you**

In higher amounts, dietary fiber can reduce absorption of vitamins, minerals, protein, and calories. Although most of us consider not absorbing calories a good thing, consult you doctor if you are taking any medications or prescribed vitamin supplements in case the flaxseed could hinder their absorption.

101. **The gas factor**

Fermentation of dietary fiber by bacteria in the large intestine can produce gas. There's no pretty way to say it, but sometimes an increase of fiber in one's diet can encourage abdominal distention or flatulence. Remember, when fiber goes up, so should your fluid or water intake. And you are more likely to avoid these side effects if you increase your fiber gradually, giving your gastrointestinal tract time to adapt. You don't want to shock your system. Starting with a tablespoon of ground flaxseed a day shouldn't be a problem for most, if you aren't changing anything else in your diet at the same time. For example, you don't want to suddenly start supplementing with flaxseed at the same time that you decide to start eating a big bowl of beans and a bowl of Kellogg's All-Bran cereal every day. Fiber overload comes from too much, too fast.

3

A Muffin a Day
and Other Breakfasts

These ten muffins have three things in common: they all taste terrific, contain 50 percent less fat than store-bought muffins, and each features ground flaxseed. Muffins can be convenient, too—you can make a batch, enjoy a few fresh from the oven, then freeze the rest in Ziploc bags. Warm flaxseed muffins are only a one-minute microwave-button away. I've also included a few other breakfast recipes I think you'll enjoy.

Banana Maple Muffins

MAKES 15 REGULAR-SIZED MUFFINS

You may be surprised how nicely the flavors of banana and maple go together. The flaxseed is almost undetectable in this recipe—the little light brown flecks look like part of the banana.

⅔ cup milk

1 tablespoon white wine, cider vinegar, or rice vinegar

2⅛ cups unbleached white flour (1⅛ cups whole wheat flour and 1 cup of all purpose can be used instead of 2⅛ cups of the white flour)

Canola cooking spray

6 tablespoons ground flaxseed

2¼ teaspoons baking powder

½ teaspoon salt

3 tablespoons butter, softened

4 tablespoons light or fat-free cream cheese

½ cup granulated sugar

¼ cup maple syrup

1 egg

4 egg whites (or ½ cup egg substitute)

2 medium ripe bananas, cut into chunks

❖ Preheat oven to 350°F. Combine the milk and vinegar in a small bowl and let stand 10 minutes. Meanwhile, coat 12 regular-sized muffin cups with canola cooking spray.

❖ Add the flour, flaxseed, baking powder, and salt to a large bowl and stir with fork to blend well.

❖ In a mixing bowl, cream the butter, cream cheese, and sugar until pale and fluffy. Add the maple syrup and blend, then add the egg and egg whites one at a time, beating until smooth.

❖ On lowest speed, gradually beat in the flour mixture alternately with the milk mixture and mix just until combined. Fold in the banana chunks.

❖ Spoon into the prepared muffin cups using ¼-cup measure and bake for about 15 minutes until well risen and golden and tester inserted into center comes out relatively clean (with a few moist crumbs on it).

PER MUFFIN: 154 calories, 4 g protein, 27 g carbohydrate, 3.5 g fat (3.3 g saturated fat, 1.6 g monounsaturated fat, 1 g polyunsaturated fat), 21 mg cholesterol, 2 g fiber, 365 mg sodium. Calories from fat: 27 percent. Omega-3 fatty acids = .6 Omega-6 fatty acids = .3 Weight Watchers Winning Points = 3

Orange-Carrot Muffins

MAKES 11 REGULAR-SIZED MUFFINS

❧

You'll want two of these for a reasonably sized breakfast or snack—this serving will provide a tablespoon of flaxseed. I often add pecans to this recipe, which complements the delightful orange flavor, but please note that they add about 36 calories and 3.6 grams of fat per muffin.

Canola cooking spray

¾ cup unbleached flour

¼ cup plus 2 tablespoons ground flaxseed

¼ cup plus 2 tablespoons oat bran

½ cup dark brown sugar, packed

1 teaspoon baking soda

1 teaspoon baking powder

¼ teaspoon salt

1 teaspoon ground cinnamon

1 cup grated carrots, packed (about 1½
   whole carrots)

½ cup chopped pecans (optional)

½ cup orange juice

⅓ cup fat-free or light sour cream

1 large egg

2 large egg whites

1 teaspoon vanilla extract

1 tablespoon canola oil

Zest (finely grated peel) from 1 orange

❖ Preheat oven to 350°F. Coat 11 muffin cups with canola cooking spray or use paper liners; set pan aside.

❖ Put the flour, flaxseed, oat bran, brown sugar, baking soda, baking powder, salt, cinnamon, carrots, and pecans (if desired) into a large mixing bowl and mix well.

❖ In another bowl, mix the orange juice, sour cream, egg and egg whites, vanilla extract, canola oil, and orange zest until well blended.

❖ Add egg mixture to dry ingredients and mix until just combined.

❖ Fill each muffin cup with ¼ cup of batter. Bake until tester inserted into center comes out clean, about 15 minutes.

PER MUFFIN: 170 calories, 5 g protein, 24 g carbohydrate, 6.5 g fat (.7 g saturated fat, 3.2 g monounsaturated fat, 2.5 g polyunsaturated fat), 20 mg cholesterol, 3 g fiber, 242 mg sodium. Calories from fat: 32 percent. Omega-3 fatty acids = 1 g Omega-6 fatty acids = 1.7 g Weight Watchers Winning Points = 3

Raisin Bran Flaxseed Muffins

MAKES 18 REGULAR-SIZED MUFFINS

Raisin bran is one of my favorite breakfast cereals, but these muffins make it taste even better because I add buttermilk and maple syrup, and are even more nutritious due to the added ground flaxseed, whole wheat flour, and canola oil.

Canola cooking spray

½ cup ground flaxseed

½ cup whole wheat flour

1½ cups unbleached white flour

1¼ cups sugar

2½ teaspoons baking soda

1 teaspoon salt

3 cups raisin bran cereal

2 cups low-fat buttermilk

¼ cup canola oil

¼ cup maple syrup

1 large egg

2 egg whites

❖ Preheat oven to 425°F and coat 18 muffin cups with canola cooking spray.

❖ Combine flaxseed, flours, sugar, baking soda, and salt in a large mixing bowl and beat on low to blend well. Add raisin bran and beat on low speed until just blended in.

❖ Combine buttermilk, oil, maple syrup, egg, and egg whites in another bowl and whisk with fork to blend well. Pour into dry ingredients and beat on low speed just to blend.

❖ Spoon ¼ cup batter into each prepared muffin cup and bake until tester inserted into center of muffins comes out clean, about 15 minutes. Transfer to rack and cool.

PER MUFFIN: 210 calories, 5 g protein, 38 g carbohydrates, 5 g fat (.6 g saturated fat, 2.3 g monounsaturated fat, 1.9 g polyunsaturated fat), 13 mg cholesterol, 3 g fiber, 403 mg sodium. Calories from fat: 21 percent. Omega-3 fatty acids = 1 g Omega-6 fatty acids = .9 g Weight Watchers Winning Points = 4

Caramel Apple Muffins

MAKES 12 REGULAR-SIZED MUFFINS

Instead of eating apple-flavored breakfast cereals with little or no fiber or apples, try making a batch of these moist Caramel Apple Muffins. Just two will give you four grams of fiber, which is a lot. And the caramel sweetener makes them totally delicious.

Canola cooking spray

¼ cup canola oil

½ cup fat-free or light sour cream

½ cup sugar

¼ cup caramel topping (from jar)

1 large egg

2 tablespoons egg substitute or 1 egg
   white

½ cup unbleached white flour

¼ cup whole wheat flour

⅓ cup rolled oats

6 tablespoons ground flaxseed

1 teaspoon ground cinnamon

½ teaspoon baking soda

¼ teaspoon ground nutmeg

¼ teaspoon salt

2 cups finely chopped apples,
   packed—peeled or not peeled
   depending on preference (cut about
   2 apples into thin slices, toss core,
   then finely chop the slices)

❖ Preheat oven to 350°F. Thickly coat muffin pan with canola cooking spray, then lightly flour each muffin cup, or use muffin papers.

❖ Combine oil, sour cream, sugar, and caramel topping in mixing bowl. Beat until well blended. Add egg and egg substitute or egg white, and beat until the mixture thickens slightly.

❖ Add dry ingredients (white and whole wheat flour, oats, flaxseed, cinnamon, baking soda, nutmeg, and salt) to food processor and pulse for about eight seconds until mixture is blended and oats have been processed into smaller pieces. Add dry mixture to the batter in mixer and beat on low just until blended. Stir chopped apples gently into batter with a spoon.

❖ Pour about ¼ cup of batter into each muffin cup and bake in center of oven until center of muffin springs back when gently pressed, about 15 minutes.

PER MUFFIN: 186 calories, 4 g protein, 29 g carbohydrate, 6.4 g fat (.7 g saturated fat, 3.2 g monounsaturated fat, 2.5 g polyunsaturated fat), 19 mg cholesterol, 3 g fiber, 144 mg sodium. Calories from fat: 31 percent. Omega-3 fatty acids = 1.2 g Omega-6 fatty acids = 1.3 g Weight Watchers Winning Points = 4

Pumpkin Apple Streusel Muffins

MAKES 18 REGULAR SIZED MUFFINS

∽

These might sound like Halloween muffins to you, but I love to make these all year round. The apple in the muffins and the streusel topping complement the pumpkin perfectly.

Canola cooking spray

1 cup whole wheat flour

1 cup unbleached or all-purpose flour

½ cup ground flaxseed

1 cup white sugar

1 tablespoon pumpkin pie spice

1 teaspoon baking soda

½ teaspoon salt

1 egg, lightly beaten

¼ cup egg substitute or 2 egg whites

1 cup canned pumpkin puree

¼ cup canola oil

7 tablespoons reduced-calorie pancake
      syrup or maple syrup

2 cups finely chopped peeled and
      cored apple (about 2 apples)

Streusel Topping:

2 tablespoons unbleached or all-
      purpose flour

¼ cup white sugar

½ teaspoon ground cinnamon

1 tablespoon melted butter

❖ Preheat oven to 350°F and lightly coat 18 muffin cups with canola cooking spray or use paper liners.

❖ In a large bowl, blend together 2 cups flour, flaxseed, 1½ cups sugar, pumpkin pie spice, baking soda, and salt. In a mixing bowl, beat together egg, egg substitute or egg whites, pumpkin, canola oil, and syrup. Add flour mixture to mixing bowl, beating on low just until blended. Fold (or beat in on low speed) the finely chopped apples. Spoon batter into prepared muffin cups.

❖ In a small bowl, mix together 2 tablespoons flour, ¼ cup sugar, and ½ teaspoon cinnamon. Drizzle melted butter over the top and blend with fork until the mixture resembles coarse crumbs. Sprinkle topping evenly over muffin batter using a measuring teaspoon.

❖ Bake until toothpick inserted into muffin comes out clean, about 35 minutes.

PER MUFFIN: 169 calories, 3 g protein, 29 g carbohydrate, 4.7 g fat (.8 g saturated fat, 2.4 g monounsaturated fat, 1.8 g polyunsaturated fat), 13 mg cholesterol, 3 g fiber, 161 mg sodium. Calories from fat: 25 percent. Omega-3 fatty acids = 1 g Omega-6 fatty acids = .9 g Weight Watchers Winning Points = 3

Banana Chocolate Chip Muffins

MAKES 12 REGULAR-SIZED MUFFINS

This recipe makes wonderful mini chocolate chip muffins when you use the mini semi-sweet chocolate chips. I like to spread my chocolate around and with mini chocolate chips, a little goes a longer way.

Canola cooking spray

1⅛ cups all-purpose flour

6 tablespoons ground flaxseed

⅔ cup sugar

1½ teaspoons baking powder

¼ teaspoon salt

1 cup mashed extra ripe bananas
   (about 2 large or 3 medium)

1 large egg

¼ cup (½ stick) butter, melted

¼ cup fat-free or light sour cream

2 teaspoons vanilla extract

¼ cup low-fat milk

½ cup mini semi-sweet chocolate
   chips (or regular sized)

❖ Preheat oven to 350°F. Line 12 muffin cups with foil muffin liners or spray muffin cups with canola cooking spray.

❖ Add flour, flaxseed, sugar, baking powder, and salt to 8-cup measure and stir with fork to blend.

❖ Add mashed bananas, egg, melted butter, sour cream, vanilla extract, and milk to mixing bowl. Beat on medium until well blended. Add dry ingredients to banana mixture while beating on low speed just until blended (do not overmix).

❖ Stir in chocolate chips.

❖ Use ⅓-cup measure to fill each muffin cup about ¾ full. Bake muffins until tops are pale golden and tester inserted into center comes out with some melted chocolate attached but no crumbs (about 30 to 32 minutes). Transfer muffins to rack and let cool.

PER MUFFIN: 199 calories, 3.5 g protein, 30.5 g carbohydrate, 7.5 g fat (4 g saturated fat, 2.3 g monounsaturated fat, 1.2 g poly-unsaturated fat), 29 mg cholesterol, 2.5 g fiber, 162 mg sodium. Calories from fat: 34 percent. Omega-3 fatty acids = .8 g Omega-6 fatty acids = .4 g. Weight Watchers Winning Points = 4

Blueberry Oat Bran Streusel Muffins

MAKES 12 MUFFINS

ॐ

Your typical 4-ounce bakery-type blueberry muffin contains 420 calories, 22 grams of fat, <1 gram of fiber, and 8½ teaspoons of sugar. By making a few ingredient adjustments, we can turn this blueberry muffin into a Blueberry Oat Bran Muffin that contains a high-fiber, whole-grain cereal plus ground flaxseed, and almost a full fruit serving per muffin, and that is much lower in total fat, saturated fat, and calories.

Canola cooking spray

1½ cups fresh or frozen blueberries

1 tablespoon flour (optional)

⅓ cup oat bran

6 tablespoons ground flaxseed

1⅓ cups unbleached flour

2 teaspoons baking powder

½ teaspoon salt

2 tablespoons canola margarine

⅓ cup light corn syrup

⅓ cup granulated sugar

1 egg

2 egg whites

1 teaspoon vanilla extract

¼ teaspoon grated dried lemon peel
   (or 1 teaspoon fresh lemon zest)

½ cup milk (low-fat or whole)

Streusel Topping:

3 tablespoons unbleached flour

3 tablespoons sugar

½ teaspoon ground cinnamon

2 tablespoons butter or canola margarine

❖ Preheat oven to 375°F. Line 12 muffin cups and spray lightly with canola cooking spray if desired.

❖ Add 3 tablespoons flour, 3 tablespoons sugar, and ½ teaspoon cinnamon to small bowl and blend well. Cut in 2 tablespoons butter with fork until mixture resembles coarse crumbs; set aside.

❖ In small bowl sprinkle 1 tablespoon flour over blueberries if desired (to keep the blueberries from turning the batter "purple"); set aside.

❖ Combine oat bran, flaxseed, 1⅓ cups flour, 2 teaspoons baking powder and ½ teaspoon salt in medium bowl.

❖ In mixer bowl, beat 2 tablespoons canola margarine, ⅓ cup light corn syrup, and ⅓ cup sugar at medium speed until light and fluffy. Add egg and egg whites, beating until smooth. Add vanilla and lemon peel.

❖ On lowest speed beat in dry ingredients, alternately with milk, beating just until blended (do not overmix). Fold blueberries into the batter gently.

❖ Spoon ¼ cup of batter into prepared cups. Sprinkle with streusel topping. Bake about 20 minutes or until toothpick inserted into center of muffin comes out clean. Cool in pans on wire rack.

PER SERVING: 206 calories, 5 g protein, 36 g carbohydrate, 5.5 g fat (.9 g saturated fat, 2.5 g monounsaturated fat, 2.2 g polyunsaturated fat), 18 mg cholesterol, 3 g fiber, 242 mg sodium. Calories from fat: 26 percent. Omega-3 fatty acids = .8 g Omega-6 fatty acids = .5 g. Weight Watchers Winning Points = 4

Fruity Flaxseed Muffins

MAKES 12 MUFFINS

ॐ

These high-flax muffins really do taste better than they sound, and they are full of flavor and moistness.

Canola cooking spray

½ cup crushed pineapple with juice
   (crushed pineapple canned in juice)

½ cup finely chopped apples

⅛ cup canola oil

1 large egg, beaten lightly

1 cup fat-free sour cream

¼ cup dark molasses

½ cup raisins

1¼ cup unbleached flour

½ cup whole wheat flour

1 teaspoon baking powder

1 teaspoon baking soda

¼ teaspoon salt

¾ cup ground flaxseed

❖ Preheat oven to 400°F. Line pan with muffin papers. Coat inside of papers with a quick squirt of canola cooking spray.

❖ In large bowl with electric mixer, cream together the pineapple with juice, apples, canola oil, egg, egg whites, sour cream, and molasses until mixture is light and fluffy. Stir in raisins.

❖ In a bowl, whisk together flours, baking powder, baking soda, salt, and flaxseed.

❖ Beating on low speed, add flaxseed mixture to sour cream mixture just until combined (batter will be a little lumpy). Spoon batter by ¼ cupfuls into prepared muffin pan.

❖ Bake in center of preheated oven for about 20 minutes or until muffins are golden brown and springy to the touch.

PER MUFFIN: 194 calories, 5 grams protein, 31 g carbohydrate, 5.5 g fat (.8 gram saturated fat, 2.1 g monounsaturated fat, 2.6 g polyunsaturated fat), 20 mg cholesterol, 4.2 grams fiber, 224 mg sodium. Calories from fat: 28 percent. Omega-3 fatty acids = 1.7 g Omega-6 fatty acids = .9 g. Weight Watchers Winning Points = 4

Carrot-Raisin Muffins

MAKES ABOUT 20 REGULAR-SIZED MUFFINS
OR 10 TEXAS-SIZED MUFFINS

⅓ cup canola oil

⅓ cup low-fat buttermilk

1 cup brown sugar, packed

⅓ cup pineapple juice (from drained
   crushed pineapple) or orange juice

1 large egg

3 egg whites

Canola cooking spray

1 cup unbleached flour

½ cup ground flaxseed

1 teaspoon baking soda

2 teaspoons baking powder

1 teaspoon ground cinnamon

½ teaspoon salt

½ cup chopped walnuts (optional)

8 ounce can crushed pineapple,
   drained (reserve juice if desired)

½ cup raisins

1 cup finely grated carrots

❖ Preheat oven to 350°F. Coat 20 regular-sized muffin pans (or 10 Texas-size) with canola cooking spray or muffin papers.

❖ Add oil, buttermilk, and brown sugar to mixing bowl. Beat to blend. Blend in pineapple juice, egg, and egg whites and beat until well mixed.

❖ Add flour and flaxseed to a 4-cup measure. Add baking soda, baking powder, cinnamon, and salt to the flour and stir with fork. Dump the flour mixture into the mixer with the wet ingredients and beat on low speed until blended, scraping sides of the bowl midway through.

❖ Add walnuts (if desired), pineapple, raisins, and carrots to muffin batter in mixing bowl and beat on low until blended, scraping sides of bowl midway through.

❖ Fill prepared muffins cups ¾ full with batter (about ¼ cup) and bake for about 20 to 25 minutes or until fork inserted into center of muffin comes out clean.

PER MUFFIN: 142 calories, 2.5 g protein, 22 g carbohydrate, 5 g fat (.5 g saturated fat, 2.5 g monounsaturated fat, 1.9 g polyunsaturated fat), 11 mg cholesterol, 1.5 gram fiber, 208 mg sodium. Calories from fat: 32 percent. Omega-3 fatty acids = .9 g Omega-6 fatty acids = .9 g. Weight Watchers Winning Points = 3

Lemon Glazed Mini Muffins

MAKES 24 MINI MUFFINS OR 8 SERVINGS (3 MINI MUFFINS PER SERVING)

৵

These muffins have that delicious, tart taste of lemon and they look and taste fancy enough to serve at a special brunch.

Canola cooking spray

3 tablespoons butter, softened

⅓ cup nonfat or light cream cheese

1 cup sugar

1 large egg

¼ cup egg substitute

Juice and finely chopped lemon zest
from 1 large lemon (about 3 table-
spoons of juice and 1 teaspoon
finely chopped lemon zest)

1 cup unbleached or all-purpose flour

½ cup ground golden flaxseed (golden
flax works best in this recipe)

1 teaspoon baking powder

½ teaspoon salt

½ cup low-fat milk

Lemon Glaze:

Juice and finely chopped lemon zest
from 2 lemons

⅓ cup granulated sugar

❖ Preheat oven to 350° F. Coat mini muffin cups with canola cooking spray.

❖ Blend butter and cream cheese together with mixer. Cream butter mixture and sugar together with mixer. Beat in egg and then egg substitute. Beat in lemon juice and zest.

❖ In another bowl, blend dry ingredients together (flour, flaxseed, baking powder, and salt). Add half of flour mixture to butter mixture, then half of milk. Add in remaining flour mixture, then remaining milk.

❖ Fill mini muffin cups almost full. Bake about 10 to 12 minutes or until middle springs back when pressed gently with finger. While muffins are baking, blend lemon glaze ingredients together. Poke the top of each muffin with toothpick or fork. Pour lemon glaze over muffins, using a ½-teaspoon measuring spoon, until it all soaks in. Let stand an hour or so.

PER 3 MINI MUFFINS: 290 calories, 7 g protein, 49 g carbohydrates, 8 g fat (3.3 g saturated fat, 2.1 g monounsaturated fat, 2.1 g polyunsaturated fat), 40 mg cholesterol, 3 g fiber, 337 mg sodium. Calories from fat: 25 percent. Omega-3 fatty acids = 1.5 g Omega-6 fatty acids = .5 g. Weight Watchers Winning Points = 6

Blueberry Buttermilk Pancakes

MAKES 4 SERVINGS (3 PANCAKES EACH)

ༀ

Pancakes are one of my favorite breakfasts and these yummy-tasting pancakes come out light and fluffy every time.

Canola cooking spray

1 cup flour

1 teaspoon baking powder

½ teaspoon baking soda

¼ teaspoon salt

1 tablespoon sugar

1 large lightly beaten egg

1¼ cups buttermilk

1 tablespoon unsalted butter, melted (canola margarine can also be used)

1 tablespoon maple syrup

1 teaspoon vanilla extract

1 cup fresh or frozen blueberries

¼ cup ground flaxseed (golden flax will hide better in this recipe)

❖ Add flour, baking powder, baking soda, salt, and sugar to mixing bowl. Beat on low to blend dry ingredients well.

❖ Add egg, buttermilk, melted butter, and maple syrup to mixing bowl and beat on low to blend (there will still be some small lumps). Let batter rest 10 minutes.

❖ Fold in blueberries and flaxseed.

❖ Heat a skillet to about 350°F or, if you're using a frying pan over a stove, heat nonstick pan to medium-low. Once a water droplet bounces around on it, your pan is ready.

❖ Pour batter by ¼ cupfuls on skillet coated with canola cooking spray, if desired. When bubbles form on top, check bottom to see if lightly browned, then flip pancakes over to cook other side.

❖ Repeat step 4 until all the batter is used.

PER SERVING: 260 calories, 9 g protein, 39 g carbohydrate, 7.5 g fat (2.8 g saturated fat, 2.1 g monounsaturated fat, 2.2 g polyunsaturated fat), 64 mg cholesterol, 4 grams fiber, 553 mg sodium. Calories from fat: 26 percent. Omega-3 fatty acids = 1.6 g Omega-6 fatty acids = .7 g. Weight Watchers Winning Points = 5
NOTE: Any pancake toppings would be additoinal to the nutrient analysis.

Mock Coco's Breakfast Burrito

MAKES 2 BURRITOS

‍‍‍‍‍‍‍‍‍‍‍‍‍‍‍‍‍‍‍‍

In this recipe, I did the unthinkable—I used all egg substitute instead of two eggs. When lightening up a mostly egg dish I usually use half real eggs and half egg whites or egg substitute. But because all the other ingredients being added to this breakfast dish contain beaucoup fat—sautéed vegetables, sausage, and bacon, cheese, sour cream, and avocado—I figured we could get away with 100 percent egg substitute. If you can't bring yourself to do this, just use ¼ cup egg substitute mixed with one large egg. The garnish of avocado, more salsa, and sour cream is optional. Adding ¼ avocado, sliced, to the burrito will add 81 calories and 7 grams fat (only 1 of the grams is from saturated fat) per serving.

Canola oil cooking spray

¼ cup chopped onion

½ cup chopped bell pepper

½ cup egg substitute (or use 1 large egg
   beaten with 2 egg whites if desired)

3 ounces turkey breakfast sausage or Jimmy
   Dean Light Sausage (50% less fat), crumbled
   up and cooked over medium heat until
   nicely browned and cooked through, or 3
   strips turkey bacon, cooked till crisp and
   broken into small bits

⅛ cup bottled or fresh salsa ("mild" or "hot"
   depending on your preference)

2 tablespoons ground flaxseed

¼ cup reduced fat cheddar cheese

2 9-inch flour tortillas (approx. 68 grams weight
   with 160 calories and .5 grams fat each)

Garnish (optional):

½ avocado, thinly sliced

¼ cup bottled or fresh salsa

¼ cup fat-free or light sour cream

❖ Add canola oil to medium nonstick frying pan over medium heat. Sauté onions and bell pepper for about 3 minutes, stirring often.

❖ Pour in the egg substitute and continue to cook, stirring frequently until eggs are cooked through, about 1 to 2 minutes. Turn off heat and stir in the cooked sausage or bacon bits, salsa, flaxseed, and cheese. Cover pan and let sit 1 to 2 minutes.

❖ Meanwhile, soften up tortillas by warming them in a microwave on high for a minute, or warming in a large, nonstick frying pan over medium heat.

❖ Spoon half of the egg mixture into the center of one of the flour tortillas and roll up like a burrito. Repeat with remaining egg mixture and tortilla. Garnish each serving with sliced avocado, and a dollop of salsa and sour cream if desired.

PER BURRITO (WITH TURKEY BACON): 342 calories, 20 g protein, 37 g carbohydrate, 12.5 g fat (3.7 g saturated fat, 3.6 g monounsaturated fat, 3.4 g polyunsaturated fat), 29 mg cholesterol, 4 grams fiber, 842 mg sodium. Calories from fat: 33 percent. Omega-3 fatty acids = 1.5 g Omega-6 fatty acids = 1.8 g. Weight Watchers Winning Points = 7
   Note: If you want the grams of fat to reduce even further, choose fat-free tortillas.

4

There's Something about Smoothies

I am addicted to smoothies. They hit the spot as a quickie breakfast, as an afternoon pick-me-up, or as a late-night treat. You can go to those smoothie shops to get your smoothie fix, but most of them don't have ground flaxseed as a possible smoothie supplement. What's the answer? M.Y.O.S—Make Your Own Smoothies.

Smoothies are a fun venue for flaxseed. What could be better than a cool, delicious Lemonade Freeze, Maui Mango Smoothie, or Mocha-ccino Freeze with a dose of ground flaxseed? With these awesome recipes, you'll never tire of sipping smoothies or getting your daily dose of flaxseed. If you are a little hesitant about adding little brown flakes to your bright orange smoothie, I suggest you use ground golden flaxseed—you won't even notice it.

Mocha-ccino Freeze

MAKES 2 SMOOTHIES

ॐ

What can I say—this creamy, chilled coffee drink is one of my favorite ways to work a dose of flaxseed into my hot summer day.

1 cup low-fat vanilla frozen yogurt or light vanilla ice cream or ice milk (nonfat or sugar-free brands can be substituted if desired)

¼ cup low-fat milk

¼ cup strong decaf coffee,* chilled (or use caffeinated if you prefer)

1 cup ice cubes

2 tablespoons ground flaxseed

❖ Add all ingredients to your blender or large food processor.

❖ Blend on highest speed until smooth, about 10 seconds. Scrape sides of blender and turn on blender for 5 seconds more.

❖ Pour into two glasses and enjoy!

PER SMOOTHIE: 157 calories, 7 g protein, 23 g carbohydrate, 4.5 g fat (1.3 g saturated fat, 1 g monounsaturated fat, 1.9 g polyunsaturated fat), 7 mg cholesterol, 2.3 g fiber, 79 mg sodium. Calories from fat: 26 percent. Omega-3 fatty acids = 1.5 g Omega-6 fatty acids = .4 g. Weight Watchers Winning Points = 3

*To make double-strength coffee, brew coffee with twice the coffee that you usually use or is indicated by your coffee maker.

Peanut Butter Cup Smoothie

ॐ

My kids went wild over this smoothie so I had to include it. In actuality, peanut butter is extremely rich in omega-6 fatty acids, which we want to avoid, but the flaxseed's healthy omega-3s counterbalance the omega-6s.

1 cup nonfat or low-fat milk

2 tablespoons creamy Reduced Fat Jif Peanut Butter (regular can be substituted)

1 cup chocolate ice milk (or similar light chocolate frozen yogurt or ice cream)

2 tablespoons cocoa powder (unsweetened)

1 to 2 cups ice cubes

2 tablespoons ground flaxseed

❖ Add all ingredients to your blender or large food processor.

❖ Blend on highest speed until smooth, about 10 seconds. Scrape sides of blender and turn on blender for 5 seconds more.

❖ Pour into two glasses and enjoy!

PER SMOOTHIE: 292 calories, 14.5 g protein, 37.5 g carbohydrate, 9.5 g fat (3.2 g saturated fat, 1.4 g monounsaturated fat, 1.9 g polyunsaturated fat), 9 mg cholesterol, 5.5 g fiber, 245 mg sodium. Calories from fat: 29 percent. Omega-3 fatty acids = 1.5 g Omega-6 fatty acids = .4 g. Weight Watchers Winning Points = 6

Blue-Raspberry Smoothie

MAKES 2 SMOOTHIES

ﾐ

There's something about blueberries, bananas, and raspberries that just go together really well in a smoothie.

1 cup frozen blueberries

1 banana (if you aren't crazy about bananas, use ½ banana instead)

1 cup raspberry sorbet

1 cup vanilla soymilk (i.e., White Wave Silk brand) (regular, low-, or nonfat milk can also be used)

2 tablespoons ground flaxseed (golden flax will hide better in this recipe)

about 2 cups ice cubes

❖ Add all ingredients to your blender or large food processor.

❖ Blend on highest speed until smooth, about 10 seconds. Scrape sides of blender and turn on blender for 5 seconds more.

❖ Pour into two glasses and enjoy!

PER SMOOTHIE (WITHOUT SUBSTITUTION): 330 calories, 6 g protein, 69 g carbohydrate, 5.5 g fat (.7 g saturated fat, .7 g monounsaturated fat, 2 g polyunsaturated fat), 0 mg cholesterol, 8 g fiber, 73 mg sodium. Calories from fat: 15 percent. Omega-3 fatty acids = 1.6 g Omega-6 fatty acids = .5 g. Weight Watchers Winning Points = 6

Strawberry-Banana-Fana Smoothie

MAKES 3 SMOOTHIES

The most popular smoothie flavor at my neighborhood smoothie shop is none other than your basic strawberry-banana smoothie. So here's my flaxseed-enhanced version.

1 cup apple juice (regular or sparkling)

2 cups frozen (unsweetened) or fresh
strawberries, packed

2 small bananas or 1 large, sliced

2 cups vanilla nonfat or low-fat frozen
yogurt or light ice cream

3 tablespoons ground flaxseed (golden
flax will hide better in this recipe)

❖ Add all ingredients to your blender or large food processor.

❖ Blend on highest speed until smooth, about 10 seconds. Scrape sides of blender and turn on blender for 5 seconds more.

❖ Pour into three glasses and enjoy!

PER SMOOTHIE: 300 calories, 9.5 g protein, 61 g carbohydrate, 3 g fat (.5 g saturated fat, .7 g monounsaturated fat, 2.1 g polyunsaturated fat), 2 mg cholesterol, 6.5 g fiber, 92 mg sodium. Calories from fat: 10 percent. Omega-3 fatty acids = 1.6 g Omega-6 fatty acids = .5 g. Weight Watchers Winning Points = 5

50/50 Bar Smoothie

MAKES 2 SMOOTHIES

I vividly remember looking forward to Dreyer's 50/50 Bars—orange sorbet and vanilla ice cream—on hot summer days. Here is that delicious combination of tastes transformed into a smoothie.

¾ cup fresh orange segments or mandarin oranges, drained (canned)*

1 cup orange juice (preferably calcium fortified)

1½ cups light vanilla ice cream, or nonfat or low-fat frozen yogurt

½ teaspoon vanilla extract (optional)

2 tablespoons ground flaxseed (golden flax will hide better in this recipe)

1–2 cups ice cubes

*If you are using the canned mandarin oranges, an 11-ounce can, drained, will give you about ¾ cup

❖ Add all ingredients to your blender or large food processor.

❖ Blend on highest speed until smooth, about 10 seconds. Scrape sides of blender and turn on blender for 5 seconds more.

❖ Pour into two glasses and enjoy!

PER SMOOTHIE (USING LIGHT ICE CREAM): 323 calories, 8 g protein, 50 g carbohydrate, 9 g fat (4 g saturated fat, .6 g monounsaturated fat, 1.9 g polyunsaturated fat), 52 mg cholesterol, 4.2 g fiber, 71 mg sodium. Calories from fat: 25 percent. Omega-3 fatty acids = 1.5 g Omega-6 fatty acids = .4 g. Weight Watchers Winning Points = 6

Maui Mango Smoothie

MAKES 2 SMOOTHIES

ॐ

I went to Hawaii to celebrate my fortieth birthday and I must have had a mango smoothie poolside each and every day I was there. I've been hooked ever since.

1 cup apricot mango nectar (like Kern's brand)

2 cups mango pieces, fresh or bottled

1 cup vanilla nonfat or low-fat frozen yogurt or light vanilla ice cream

2 cups ice cubes

2 tablespoons ground flaxseed (golden flax will hide better in this recipe)

❖ Add all ingredients to your blender or large food processor.

❖ Blend on highest speed until smooth, about 10 seconds. Scrape sides of blender and turn on blender for 5 seconds more.

❖ Pour into two glasses and enjoy!

PER SMOOTHIE: 314 calories, 7.5 g protein, 68 g carbohydrate, 3.5 g fat (.5 g saturated fat, .8 g monounsaturated fat, 1.9 g polyunsaturated fat), 1 mg cholesterol, 6 g fiber, 74 mg sodium. Calories from fat: 10 percent. Omega-3 fatty acids = 1.5 g Omega-6 fatty acids = .4 g. Weight Watchers Winning Points = 6

Lemonade Freeze

ॐ

This smoothie reminds me of those lemonade freezes you can buy at county fairs or amusement parks. You can easily make these lower in sugar calories by using sugar-free lemonade and reduced-calorie sorbet. The yogurt adds some creaminess and a little boost of calcium and protein.

2 cups reduced calorie lemon sorbet
(or regular lemon sorbet)

1 cup sugar-free lemonade

6 ounces low-fat lime or key lime
yogurt

2 cups ice

3 tablespoons ground flaxseed (golden
flax will hide better in this recipe)

❖ Add all ingredients to your blender or large food processor.

❖ Blend on highest speed until smooth, about 10 seconds. Scrape sides of blender and turn on blender for 5 seconds more.

❖ Pour into three glasses and enjoy!

PER SMOOTHIE: 130 calories, 4 g protein, 20 g carbohydrate, 3.4 g fat (.6 g saturated fat, .5 monounsaturated fat, 1.8 g poly-unsaturated fat), 3 mg cholesterol, 2.5 g fiber, 68 mg sodium. Calories from fat: 24 percent. Omega-3 fatty acids = 1.5 g Omega-6 fatty acids = .35 g. Weight Watchers Winning Points = 2

Purely Peach Smoothie

MAKES 2 SMOOTHIES

ↄↄ

This is for all you peach lovers out there. The only thing that isn't peachy about this smoothie is the flaxseed.

¾ cup peach nectar (like Kern's brand)

1 cup fresh, canned (in juice), or frozen
    peaches

6 ounces low-fat peach yogurt

2 tablespoons ground flaxseed

2 cups ice cubes

❖ Add all ingredients to your blender or large food processor.

❖ Blend on highest speed until smooth, about 10 seconds. Scrape sides of blender and turn on blender for 5 seconds more.

❖ Pour into two glasses and enjoy!

PER SMOOTHIE: 216 calories, 6 g protein, 42 g carbohydrate, 3.8 g fat (.8 g saturated fat, .6 g monounsaturated fat, 1.9 g polyunsaturated fat), 6 mg cholesterol, 4.5 g fiber, 65 mg sodium. Calories from fat: 16 percent. Omega-3 fatty acids = 1.5 g Omega-6 fatty acids = .4 g. Weight Watchers Winning Points = 4

Piña Colada Smoothie

MAKES 2 SMOOTHIES

ॐ

This one is my sister's favorite—I whipped up this recipe as a way to inspire her to get her flaxseed dose for the day, and it worked.

½ cup crushed pineapple canned in
    juice (including juice)

¼ to ½ teaspoon coconut extract

⅓ cup soy milk (I use the White Wave
    Silk brand) or low-fat milk

1 small banana or 6 ounces low-fat
    vanilla yogurt

⅔ cup vanilla nonfat frozen yogurt or
    light vanilla ice cream

2 tablespoons ground flaxseed

1–2 cups ice cubes

❖ Add all ingredients to your blender or large food processor.

❖ Blend on highest speed until smooth, about 10 seconds. Scrape sides of blender and turn on blender for 5 seconds more.

❖ Pour into two glasses and enjoy!

PER SMOOTHIE: 272 calories, 9 g protein, 42.5 g carbohydrate, 7 g fat (2.9 g saturated fat, .6 g monounsaturated fat, 1.8 g polyunsaturated fat), 32 mg cholesterol, 3 g fiber, 118 mg sodium. Calories from fat: 25 percent. Omega-3 fatty acids = 1.5 g Omega-6 fatty acids = .4 g. Weight Watchers Winning Points = 5

Cranberry Cooler

༄

Taste this smoothie before you pour it into cups. If it tastes a little too tart, add a tablespoon of granulated sugar or honey and give it another whirl. You can find bags of cranberries in the frozen fruit section of many grocery stores these days.

1 cup reduced-calorie cranberry juice cocktail

1 cup frozen cranberries (fresh can also be used)

1 cup raspberry sorbet or sherbet

6 ounces low-fat vanilla yogurt

2 tablespoons ground flaxseed

1–2 cups ice cubes

❖ Add all ingredients to your blender or large food processor.

❖ Blend on highest speed until smooth, about 10 seconds. Scrape sides of blender and turn on blender for 5 seconds more.

❖ Pour into two glasses and enjoy!

PER SMOOTHIE: 296 calories, 6 g protein, 61 g carbohydrate, 3.8 g fat (.8 g saturated fat, .6 g monounsaturated fat, 1.9 g polyunsaturated fat), 6 mg cholesterol, 6.3 g fiber, 63 mg sodium. Calories from fat: 12 percent. Omega-3 fatty acids = 1.5 g Omega-6 fatty acids = .4 g. Weight Watchers Winning Points = 5

Chocolate-Raspberry Smoothie

MAKES 3 SMOOTHIES

ॐ

If your favorite chocolate truffle flavor is raspberry, this is the smoothie for you. While you are enjoying this decadent-tasting drink, chew on the fact that each serving contains almost ten grams of fiber.

2 cups frozen raspberries (fresh raspberries can also be used)

2 cups low-fat chocolate fudge brownie frozen yogurt (or similar)

1 cup vanilla soy milk* (like the White Wave Silk brand) or low-fat milk

3 tablespoons ground flaxseed

1–2 cups of ice

❖ Add all ingredients to your blender or large food processor.

❖ Blend on highest speed until smooth, about 10 seconds. Scrape sides of blender and turn on blender for 5 seconds more.

❖ Pour into three glasses and enjoy!

* If you don't want to use soy milk, use non-fat or low-fat milk and add 1 teaspoon of vanilla extract.

PER SMOOTHIE: 260 calories, 11 g protein, 43 g carbohydrate, 6.5 g fat (1.8 g saturated fat, 1.3 g monounsaturated fat, 2.2 g polyunsaturated fat), 6 mg cholesterol, 9.8 g fiber, 109 mg sodium. Calories from fat: 22 percent. Omega-3 fatty acids = 1.6 g Omega-6 fatty acids = .6 g. Weight Watchers Winning Points = 5

Apricot-Orange Smoothie

MAKES 2 SMOOTHIES

ॐ

15-ounce can of chunky ready-cut apricots in light syrup

6 ounces vanilla yogurt (custard-style
works great)

1 cup orange juice (calcium fortified
orange juice is now available in car-
tons)

2 cups ice cubes

2 tablespoons ground flaxseed

❖ Add all ingredients to your blender or large food
processor.

❖ Blend on highest speed until smooth, about 10
seconds. Scrape sides of blender and turn on
blender for 5 seconds more.

❖ Pour into two glasses and enjoy!

Per smoothie: 193 calories, 7.5 g protein, 33 g carbohydrate, 4 g fat
(.9 g saturated fat, .9 monounsaturated fat, 1.9 g polyunsaturated
fat), 4 mg cholesterol, 4 g fiber, 72 mg sodium. Calories from fat: 19
percent. Omega-3 fatty acids = 1.5 g Omega-6 fatty acids = .4 g.
Weight Watchers Winning Points = 3

5

Bread Therapy

Bakers have been adding flaxseed to their bread for hundreds of years, and I say if it ain't broke, don't fix it. Adding ground flaxseed to bread seems like a no-brainer since we know that if we don't grind up the flaxseed, the seeds pass through our system undigested and unutilized. But I was shocked to discover that several commercial bakeries making five- or nine-grain breads containing flaxseed actually use whole and not ground flaxseed.

The trick is to add enough flaxseed to your bread recipe so that you get your daily dose in two or three slices, but not add so much flaxseed that the bread won't rise as it should. What you need to do is to decrease the flour, oats, or wheat bran accordingly to compensate for the amount of flaxseed added. In these bread recipes, I've added the flaxseed two ways; in the bread dough itself, or as a topping or swirl in the bread.

Cinnamon Swirl Bread

MAKES 2 LOAVES (10 SLICES EACH)

᠔

What can I say, my girls like their bread white and airy. If it's got brown flecks of anything in it—other than chocolate, that is—they most likely aren't going to eat it. To get around this, I decided to make a white bread dough, then use brown sugar in the swirl so I could hide the ground flaxseed in the cinnamon swirl part, and it worked like a charm. This recipe gives you enough dough to make two loaves, so you can even make one loaf with raisins and flaxseed in the cinnamon-sugar swirl and one loaf without. This bread is great warm from the oven or stored for several days in a sealed bag and used for toast.

Bread Dough:

2 cups warm water (100–110° F)

2 tablespoons powdered milk

2 tablespoons honey

2 tablespoons canola oil

2 teaspoons salt

1 packet active dry yeast (about 2½ teaspoons)

6 cups bread flour, plus more for dusting (all-purpose can also be used)

Filling:

¾ cup dark brown sugar, firmly packed

7 teaspoons ground cinnamon

½ cup ground flaxseed (¼ cup per loaf)

¼ cup egg substitute (1 beaten egg can also be used)

2 tablespoons butter or canola margarine, melted

1 cup baking raisins (½ cup per loaf) (optional)

Canola cooking spray

❖ Add bread dough ingredients to the bread machine pan in the order recommended by the manufacturer (for my machine it went in this order: water, powdered milk, honey, canola oil, salt, then flour. Make a well in the center of the flour and add the yeast.)

❖ Press the DOUGH button (or set for 1 hour and 40 minutes) and press the START button.

❖ Meanwhile, blend the brown sugar, cinnamon, and flaxseed together in a 2-cup measure with a fork; set aside.

❖ When the dough is ready, line a flat surface with wax paper and dust the surface with about ¼ cup of flour (add more if needed). Transfer the dough to the floured surface and cut it in half. Set one of the halves aside. Press or roll one of the dough balls into a 10 × 12-inch rectangle. Brush the top with half of the egg substitute then sprinkle with half of the cinnamon sugar mixture and drizzle half of the butter over the top. Rub the surface with the back of a spoon to blend butter and sugar mixture. Sprinkle ½ cup of raisins over the top if desired.

❖ Start at the short end and roll up dough tightly, and pinch together along the crease and at the ends. Transfer the bread dough (seam side down) to a 9 × 5-inch loaf pan that has been coated with canola cooking spray (spray the top of the bread dough with canola cooking spray too, if desired) and cover loosely with plastic wrap.

❖ Repeat steps with remaining dough and filling. Let loaves rise in a warm place for 45 minutes to 1 hour (or let sit overnight in the refrigerator).

❖ Preheat oven to 425° F and bake loaves for 15 minutes. Lower heat to 400° F and bake 15 to 20 minutes more or until bread tests done in the center. Remove from oven and cool on a wire rack for at least 30 minutes before slicing.

If you don't have a bread machine:

1. Add ¼ cup of the warm water, 1 tablespoon of the honey, and the packet of yeast together in a small bowl and stir with fork; set in a warm place to proof or get bubbly (about 10 minutes).

2. Then in a mixer bowl by hand or with an electric mixer, combine the remaining bread dough ingredients (except the flour). Stir the yeast mixture in. Slowly beat or stir in the flour.

3. On a lightly floured flat surface, knead the bread dough until elastic, about 10 minutes. Place in a buttered bowl, cover with plastic wrap, and let rise in a warm place until doubled in size, about 1 hour.

4. Punch dough down and follow directions above starting with step #3.

PER SLICE: 222 calories, 6 g protein, 43 g carbohydrate, 3.5 g fat (.9 g saturated fat, 1.4 g monounsaturated fat, 1.2 g polyunsaturated fat), 3 mg cholesterol, 2.5 g fiber, 259 mg sodium. Calories from fat: 14 percent. Omega-3 fatty acids = .7 g Omega-6 fatty acids = .5 g. Weight Watchers Winning Points = 4

Herb Crescent Rolls

৵

These rolls are so good, nobody can eat just one. In fact, if you have three rolls, you will get a whole tablespoon of ground flaxseed. I converted the recipe to a bread machine—I just used the DOUGH cycle so I could shape the dough before letting it rise the second and final time. (If you don't have a bread machine, follow the directions at the bottom of the recipe.) Make a batch and freeze some in Ziploc bags. They are a perfect last-minute accompaniment to a nice bowl of soup or salad.

¼ cup warm water

1 tablespoon sugar

1 cup small curd cottage cheese, slightly warmed in the microwave

2 teaspoons dried "fine herbs" or similar herb blend

2 tablespoons snipped chives or finely chopped green onion tops

1 teaspoon salt

1 large egg (¼ cup egg substitute can also be used)

3 cups unbleached white flour (1½ cups white flour and 1½ cups whole wheat can also be used)

⅛–¼ cup ground flaxseed (golden flax works better in this recipe)

1 package active dry yeast (2 teaspoons)

½ teaspoon baking powder

2 tablespoons butter (or canola or olive oil margarine), softened

Canola cooking spray

❖ Add water, sugar, cottage cheese, fines herbs, chives, salt, egg, flour, and flaxseed to bread machine pan. Make a well in the center of the flour and add the yeast. Pour the baking powder in one of the corners of the pan. (You can also default to the order of ingredients recommended in your bread machine manual).

❖ Set your bread machine to DOUGH cycle and press START.

❖ When cycle is completed, around 1 hour and 40 minutes later, remove your dough to a lightly floured flat surface. Using a rolling pin, roll the dough into a 13- or 14-inch circle.

❖ Preheat oven to 350° F. Spray tops with canola cooking spay if desired.

❖ Spread the softened butter over the entire top of the circle using the back of a spoon and sprinkle the top evenly with the flaxseed. Cut circle into 12 triangles.

❖ Starting from the bigger end, roll each wedge into a crescent. Transfer crescents to a baking sheet coated with canola cooking spray. Let rolls rise, uncovered, for about 45 minutes or until doubled in size.

❖ Bake for 12–15 minutes or until golden brown. Serve warm.

If you don't have a bread machine:

1. Add the water, sugar, and yeast together in a small bowl and stir with a fork; set in a warm place to proof—or get bubbly, about 10 minutes.
2. Then, in a mixer bowl, combine the cottage cheese, fine herbs, chives, baking powder, salt, and egg until well blended.
3. When the yeast mixture is bubbly, stir it into the cottage cheese mixture. Stir in the flour.
4. On a lightly floured flat surface, knead the dough until elastic, about 10 minutes.
5. Place in a buttered bowl, cover with plastic wrap, and let rise in a warm place until doubled in size, about 1 hour.
6. Punch down dough and follow the directions above, starting with step 3.

PER CRESCENT ROLL (IF USING ¼ CUP FLAX PER RECIPE): 162 calories, 7 g protein, 24 g carbohydrate, 4 g fat (2 g saturated fat, .9 g monounsaturated fat, .7 g polyunsaturated fat), 26 mg cholesterol, 2 g fiber, 306 mg sodium. Calories from fat: 22 percent. Omega-3 fatty acids = .5 gram Omega-6 fatty acids = .2 gram. Weight Watchers Winning Points = 3

Honey Wheat Buttermilk Bread or Rolls

MAKES 1 LOAF (12 SLICES PER LOAF) OR 10 ROLLS

ॐ

I like to use my bread machine to make the dough and let it rise once—then I set it in my regular loaf pan and let it rise again overnight in my refrigerator. In the morning, I simply take it out and bake. It tastes great right out of the oven. This recipe also makes wonderful wheat rolls for dinner. Just take the dough out after the dough cycle is done, shape into about ten balls, and let rise on a lightly greased cookie sheet. Then bake for about fifteen minutes or until golden brown.

¼ cup honey

1 large egg, beaten (egg substitute can be substituted)

1 cup low-fat buttermilk

1¼ cups whole wheat flour

¼ cup ground flaxseed

1¾ cups white bread flour (unbleached white or all-purpose flour can be substituted)

1½ teaspoons salt

½ teaspoon ground cinnamon (optional)

3 teaspoons active dry yeast (1 packet can be used)

1 teaspoon melted butter or canola oil (optional)

1 tablespoon oats (optional)

Canola cooking spray

PER SLICE: 160 calories, 6 g protein, 30 g carbohydrate, 2 g fat, (.7 g saturated fat, .6 g monounsaturated, .5 g polyunsaturated fat), 18 mg cholesterol, 3 g fiber, 323 mg sodium. Calories from fat: 12 percent. Omega-3 fatty acids = .5 g. Omega-6 fatty acids = .3 g. Weight Watchers Winning Points = 3

❖ Add all the ingredients to the bread machine pan in the order recommended by the manufacturer. The last ingredient added is usually the yeast; make a well in the center of the flour and then add it.

❖ Set bread machine to the DOUGH cycle (usually 1 hour and 40 minutes) and press START.

❖ When the bread machine is done, remove the dough from the pan and place it in a lightly oiled loaf pan (or spray pan with canola cooking spray). Cover with plastic wrap that has been sprayed with canola cooking spray so it doesn't stick to the dough and place in the refrigerator to rise overnight, or while you work or play during the day (or let it rise in a warm place until doubled in size).

❖ Preheat oven to 350° F. Gently brush the top of the loaf with melted butter or canola oil, then sprinkle oats over the top of the loaf, if desired.

❖ Bake bread for 30 to 35 minutes or until bread tests done.

If you don't have a bread machine:

1. Warm ¼ cup of the buttermilk in a 1-cup glass measure or small bowl in the microwave (should be warm to the touch, but not too hot).
2. Stir in 1 tablespoon of the honey and the packet of yeast using a fork; set in a warm place to proof or get bubbly, about 10 minutes.
3. Then in a mixer bowl by hand or with an electric mixer, combine the rest of the honey, the egg, and the rest of the buttermilk, and the yeast mixture.
4. In a separate medium-sized bowl, stir the flours, flaxseed, salt, and cinnamon together. Slowly beat or stir in the flour mixture until completely combined.
5. On a lightly floured flat surface, knead the bread dough until elastic, about 10 minutes. Place in a buttered bowl, cover with plastic wrap, and let rise in a warm place until doubled in size, about 1 hour.
6. Punch dough down and follow directions above starting with step #3.

Pumpkin Bran/Flax Bread

MAKES 2 LOAVES (10 SLICES EACH)

☙

Are you craving some All-Bran cereal? Say no more—I'm going to do you two steps better and add some ground flaxseed and pureed pumpkin as well. This way you'll get a boost of fiber, carotenoids from the pumpkin, and a small dose of ground flaxseed. The recipe makes two loaves, so make sure you have plenty of room in your freezer.

Canola cooking spray

2½ cups unbleached flour, plus more for dusting

½ cup ground flaxseed

1½ cups shredded bran cereal (Kellogg's All Bran cereal works great)

2 teaspoons baking soda

1½ teaspoon salt

1¼ teaspoons ground cinnamon

1 teaspoon ground allspice

½ teaspoon ground nutmeg

2 teaspoons baking powder

2 eggs

½ cup egg substitute or 4 egg whites

1¾ cups sugar

¾ cup buttermilk

2 cups canned solid pack pumpkin

⅓ cup canola oil

⅓ cup reduced-calorie pancake syrup (or maple syrup)

½ cup chopped pecans (optional)

❖ Preheat oven to 325° F. Coat two 9 × 5 × 3-inch loaf pans with canola cooking spray. Dust pans lightly with flour.

❖ Combine flour, flaxseed, bran cereal, baking soda, salt, cinnamon, allspice, nutmeg, and baking powder in medium bowl; stir to blend well.

❖ Add eggs, egg substitute, or egg whites, sugar, and buttermilk in mixing bowl. Beat until blended.

❖ Add dry ingredients and beat on low to combine. Add pumpkin, canola oil, and syrup and beat on low until blended. Divide batter between prepared pans. Sprinkle ¼ cup of chopped pecans down the center of each loaf, if desired.

❖ Bake until tester inserted into center of each loaf comes out clean, about 1 hour to 1 hour and 20 minutes. Let loaves cool 10 minutes. Turn out loaves onto racks and cool completely. Loaves or slices can be wrapped tightly and frozen up to 1 month.

PER SLICE: 208 calories, 4.5 g protein, 37 g carbohydrate, 5.5 g fat (.6 g saturated fat, 2.7 g monounsaturated fat, 2 g polyunsaturated fat), 21 mg cholesterol, 3.5 g fiber, 395 mg sodium. Calories from fat: 24 percent. Omega-3 fatty acids = .9 g Omega-6 fatty acids = 1 g Weight Watchers Winning Points = 4

Raspberry Walnut Bread

MAKES 2 LOAVES (10 SLICES EACH)

౨つ

A bag of frozen raspberries will usually be just the amount you need for this recipe. Though this bread is a bit high in omega-6 fatty acids because it contains walnuts, the flaxseed benefits go a long way toward counteracting them.

Canola cooking spray

1 cup whole wheat flour

1½ cups unbleached white flour

½ cup ground flaxseed

1 teaspoon salt

1 teaspoon baking soda

3 teaspoons cinnamon

1 teaspoon baking powder

½ cup chopped walnuts

2 eggs

2 egg whites

¼ cup canola oil

⅔ cup light corn syrup

1 cup sugar (can be reduced to ⅔ cup)

2 cups raspberries, washed and well drained (fresh or frozen). Can be increased to 3 cups.

1 tablespoon vanilla extract

❖ Preheat oven to 325° F. Coat 2 regular-sized loaf pans with canola cooking spray.

❖ Add flours, flaxseed, salt, baking soda, cinnamon, and baking powder to medium-sized bowl and stir with fork to blend well; set aside.

❖ Beat eggs and egg whites with mixer; add canola oil, corn syrup, and sugar. Beat until creamy.

❖ Beat in dry ingredients on low speed until blended.

❖ Gently stir in the raspberries, vanilla, and walnuts to egg mixture.

❖ Spread evenly in 2 regular-sized loaf pans coated with canola cooking spray. Bake for 60 minutes or until tester inserted into center comes out clean.

PER SERVING: 199 calories, 4 g protein, 33 g carbohydrate, 6 g fat (.6 g saturated fat, 2.3 g monounsaturated fat, 3 g polyunsaturated fat), 10 mg cholesterol, 3 g fiber, 234 mg sodium. Calories from fat: 27 percent. Omega-3 fatty acids = 1.1 g Omega-6 fatty acids = 2 g. Weight Watchers Winning Points = 4

Challah Bread Braid

ว๖

This recipe is great because you can use challah bread to make a fancy French toast, strata (breakfast bread and egg casserole), or any other recipe calling for bread or bread cubes. Since challah bread has a distinct yellowish tint, you might want to use golden flaxseed in this recipe.

¾ cup low-fat milk, warm to the touch (microwave on high for 30–50 seconds)

1 large egg, lightly beaten

¼ cup egg substitute

2 tablespoons canola oil, butter or canola margarine

1 tablespoon honey

5 drops yellow food coloring (optional)

3 cups all-purpose flour or bread flour

½ cup ground golden flaxseed (regular flax can be used but the brownish flecks will be more obvious in the bread)

¼ cup granulated sugar

1½ teaspoons salt

1½ teaspoons active dry yeast (or 1 packet)

Brush on top:

2 tablespoons low-fat milk

❖ Add ingredients to bread machine pan in the order suggested by the manufacturer. For my machine, I added the milk, then egg and egg substitute, butter, honey, yellow food coloring if desired, flour, and flaxseed. I added the sugar on top of the flour, spooned the salt into one of the corners, and made a well in the center of the flour and added the yeast.

❖ Select the DOUGH cycle (about 1 hour and 40 minutes) and press START.

❖ When the dough cycle is finished, turn the oven on to 375° F. Then divide the dough into 3 equal parts. On a lightly floured board, roll each part into a rope about 16 inches long. Line the 3 ropes up, side by side, on a large cookie sheet. Then press the ropes together at the top end. Braid the ropes together, pressing the ends together when you reach the bottom.

❖ Brush the top generously with 2 tablespoons low-fat milk. Set the cookie sheet on top of the oven (or another warm place) and let rise about 30 minutes.

❖ Bake 35 to 45 minutes or until lightly browned and cooked throughout.

If you don't have a bread machine:

1. Warm ¼ cup of the milk in a 1-cup glass measure or small bowl in the microwave (should be warm to the touch, but not too hot).
2. Stir in the 1 tablespoon of the granulated sugar and the packet of yeast using a fork; set in a warm place to proof or get bubbly, about 10 minutes.
3. Then in a mixer bowl by hand or with an electric mixer, combine the rest of the milk, the egg, egg substitute, canola oil, honey, and yellow food coloring. Then stir in the yeast mixture.
4. In a separate medium-sized bowl, add the flour, flaxseed, and salt and stir together with a fork. Slowly beat or stir in the flour mixture until completely combined with wet ingredients.
5. On a lightly floured flat surface, knead the bread dough until elastic, about 10 minutes.
6. Place in a buttered bowl, cover with plastic wrap, and let rise in a warm place until doubled in size, about 1 hour.
7. Punch dough down and follow directions above starting with step #3.

PER SERVING: 198 calories, 7.5 g protein, 32 g carbohydrate, 4.4 g fat (.5 g saturated fat, 1.9 g monounsasturated fat, 1.6 g polyunsaturated fat), 27 mg cholesterol, 3 g fiber, 403 mg sodium. Calories from fat: 20 percent. Omega-3 fatty acids = 1.5 g Omega-6 fatty acids = .4 g. Weight Watchers Winning Points = 4

Design Your Own Flaxseed Bread

MAKES 2 LOAVES (10 SLICES EACH)

ॐ

Here are some ways to design your own flaxseed bread. Use one or a combination of two of the designer ingredients below to create the bread of your choosing. For example, a cup of chopped cherries and a cup of chopped dates will create Cherry-Date Bread, and a cup of chopped apricots and a cup of crushed pineapple will make Apricot-Pineapple Bread.

Designer Ingredients:

Use one of the following, or a mixture of the following, to equal 2 cups, except as indicated.

Apples, grated
Applesauce
Apricots, chopped
Bananas, mashed
Carrots, grated
Cherries, pitted and chopped
Dates, pitted and finely chopped
Lemons (use only ½ cup juice)
Mincemeat
Oranges, chopped
Peaches, fresh or canned, chopped
Pears, chopped
Pineapple, crushed, well drained
Prunes, chopped (use not more than 1 cup)
Pumpkin, canned
Raisins
Raspberries
Rhubarb, finely chopped
Strawberries, fresh or well drained frozen
Sweet potato or yams, grated coarsely
Yoplait yogurt, plain or flavored (or any brand you like)
Zucchini, ground or grated, well drained

Canola cooking spray

1 cup whole wheat flour

1½ cups unbleached white flour

½ cup ground flaxseed

1 teaspoon salt

1 teaspoon baking soda

3 teaspoons cinnamon

1 teaspoon baking powder

2 eggs

2 egg whites

¼ cup canola oil

⅔ cup light corn syrup

1 cup sugar

2 cups designer ingredient(s)

1 tablespoon vanilla extract

❖ Preheat oven to 325° F. Coat 2 regular-sized loaf pans with canola cooking spray.

❖ Add flours, flaxseed, salt, baking soda, cinnamon, and baking powder to medium-sized bowl and stir with a fork to blend well and set aside.

❖ Beat eggs and egg whites with mixer; add canola oil, corn syrup, and sugar. Beat until creamy.

❖ Add the designer ingredient(s) and vanilla to egg mixture.

❖ Add dry ingredients and beat until just blended.

❖ Spread evenly in 2 regular-sized loaf pans coated with canola cooking spray. Bake for 50 to 60 minutes or until tester inserted in center comes out clean.

PER SLICE (This depends on the choices of ingredients. The analysis below is for Apricot-Pineapple Bread and includes 1 cup of chopped apricots and 1 cup of crushed pineapple.) 180 calories, 3.5 g protein, 33 g carbohydrate, 4 g fat (.5 g saturated fat, 2 g monounsaturated fat, 1.7 g polyunsaturated fat), 21 mg cholesterol, 3 g fiber, 231 mg sodium. Calories from fat: 22 percent. Omega-3 fatty acids = .9 gram Omega-6 fatty acids = .8 gram. Weight Watchers Winning Points = 3

Apple Fritter Bread Braid

ک

This bread tastes as good as it looks. The sautéed apples offer a nice surprise in every bite and the cinnamon glaze tops it off perfectly.

1 tablespoon butter

3 cups diced peeled tart apples (about 2 large apples)

½ cup apple juice

2 tablespoon sugar

1 teaspoon ground cinnamon

⅔ cup sugar

4 cups unbleached flour, divided use

½ cup ground flaxseed

1 teaspoon salt

4 teaspoons active dry yeast

1 cup plus 2 tablespoons low-fat or whole milk

3 tablespoons melted butter

1 egg, lightly beaten

¼ cup egg substitute

Canola cooking spray

Apple glaze:

1½ cups powdered sugar

4 teaspoons melted butter

4 teaspoons concentrated apple juice

2–4 pinches ground cinnamon

❖ Start melting 1 tablespoon butter in large, non-stick frying pan. Add apples and sauté 3 minutes, stirring frequently. Sprinkle ½ cup apple juice, 2 tablespoons sugar, and 1 teaspoon cinnamon over the apples and simmer 3 minutes longer; set aside to cool.

❖ In large mixing bowl, combine ⅔ cup sugar, 3 cups flour, flaxseed, salt, and yeast together and set aside.

❖ In small saucepan, heat milk and 3 tablespoons butter together, stirring constantly, just until warm to the touch and butter is melted.

❖ Add milk mixture to flour mixture in large mixing bowl and beat on low for 30 seconds. Add egg and egg substitute and beat on low for 30 seconds, stopping to scrape sides of bowl. Beat on medium-high speed for 2 minutes. On low speed, beat in apple mixture. While continuing to beat on low speed, add as much of the remaining 1 cup of flour as you can.

❖ Turn dough out onto a well-floured surface and knead in enough of the remaining flour to make a moderately stiff dough, about 3 minutes.

- ❖ Shape into 2 balls and let rest 15 minutes.
- ❖ Divide each ball into 3 pieces. Roll each piece into a rope about an inch wide and 12 inches long. Press the three ropes together at one end using your hands, place it on a cookie sheet coated with canola cooking spray, then make a braid using the three ropes. Press the ends of the braid together.
- ❖ Repeat with remaining dough. Let braids rise at room temperature for an hour or in the refrigerator overnight.
- ❖ Preheat oven to 400° F.
- ❖ Bake until braids are light brown on top and cooked throughout, about 25 minutes. While the braids bake, beat the apple glaze ingredients together with an electric mixer until smooth. When the braids come out of the oven, generously coat each with icing.

PER SERVING: 270 calories, 6 g protein, 50 g carbohydrate, 5.5 g fat (2.6 g saturated fat, 1.5 g monounsaturated fat, 1.1 g polyunsaturated fat), 24 mg cholesterol, 3 g fiber, 204 mg sodium. Calories from fat: 18 percent. Omega-3 fatty acids = .8 g Omega-6 fatty acids = .3 g. Weight Watchers Winning Points = 5

Maple Oat Scones

MAKES 8 SCONES

If you like Starbucks' maple scones, you'll love this lower-fat and -calorie version—each scone comes complete with a tablespoon of ground flax.

Canola cooking spray

1¼ cups unbleached flour

½ cup ground golden flaxseed (golden works best in this recipe)

½ cup quick or old fashioned oats

2 tablespoons sugar

½ teaspoon salt

1 tablespoon baking powder

2 tablespoons reduced calorie pancake syrup or maple syrup

2½ tablespoons cold butter, cut into small pieces

1 egg

½ cup whole milk (low-fat milk or fat-free half-and-half can be substituted)

½ teaspoon maple extract (¾ teaspoon if you want a stronger maple flavor in the dough)

⅔ cup coarsely chopped pecans (a little smaller than pecan pieces but bigger than finely chopped pecans)

Maple Glaze:

1½ cups powdered sugar

½ teaspoon maple extract

5 teaspoons water

❖ Preheat oven to 425° F. Make a 9-inch circle with canola cooking spray on a thick baking sheet.

❖ Place flour, flaxseed, oats, sugar, salt, and baking powder in food processor. Pulse to mix and finely grind the oats with the flour.

❖ Add maple syrup and butter pieces to the flour mixture and pulse to blend the two well, until the butter is broken up into very small pieces.

❖ In a separate small bowl, beat the egg lightly with the milk and ½ teaspoon maple extract. Pour the milk mixture into the flour mixture in the food processor. Pulse briefly to make a dough.

❖ Place dough on well-floured surface. Sprinkle pecans over the top and knead lightly 4 times to evenly distribute the pecans. Pat dough into a 7 ½-inch circle. Cut into 8 wedges. Place wedges in a circle on prepared baking sheet about ½ inch from each other. Bake in center of oven for about 13 to 15 minutes (top will be lightly browned).

❖ While scones are baking, combine glaze ingredients in a small bowl and stir well until smooth.

Remove scones from oven to wire rack and let cool about 3 to 5 minutes. Spread glaze generously over each scone. Once glaze has dried, about 15 minutes, the scones can be served. They keep well overnight in a plastic bag.

PER SCONE: 354 calories, 6.5 g protein, 51 g carbohydrate, 15 g fat (3.6 g saturated fat, 6.2 g monounsaturated fat, 4.3 g polyunsaturated fat), 38 mg cholesterol, 4.2 g fiber, 383 mg sodium. Calories from fat: 38 percent. Omega-3 fatty acids = 1.6 g, Omega-6 fatty acids = 2.6 g. Weight Watchers Winning Points = 7

Quick Focaccia

❧

This recipe transforms Reduced Fat Bisquick into flavorful focaccia bread.

2 tablespoons olive oil

2 garlic cloves, minced or pressed

canola oil or olive oil cooking spray

3 cups Reduced Fat Bisquick baking mix

⅓ cup ground flaxseed

2 teaspoons rubbed sage or 1 teaspoon ground sage

1 cup plus 2 tablespoons low-fat milk

⅓ cup shredded Parmesan cheese

¾ teaspoon dried oregano leaves

¼ teaspoon (add ¼ more teaspoon if desired)

❖ Combine olive oil and garlic in a small cup and set aside. If possible, allow the oil to steep overnight before using.

❖ Preheat the oven to 400°F. Coat a 13 × 9-inch baking pan generously with olive oil cooking spray.

❖ In a large bowl, blend the baking mix, flaxseed, and sage. Stir in the milk until well mixed. Turn the biscuit dough into the prepared pan and pat out evenly with floured fingertips. Make indentations in the dough with your fingertips at 1-inch intervals.

❖ Spread the garlic-oil mixture evenly over the dough with your fingertips. In a small bowl, stir the Parmesan cheese, oregano, and salt together. (Or combine in a mini food processor.) Sprinkle the dough with the cheese mixture.

❖ Bake for 25 minutes, or until nicely browned on top. Cut up into rectangles and serve warm.

PER SERVING: 250 calories, 7 g protein, 36 g carbohydrate, 8 g fat (2 g saturated fat, 3.4 g monounsaturated fat, 1.5 g polyunsaturated fat), 4 mg cholesterol, 2.1 g fiber, 671 mg sodium. Calories from fat: 30 percent. Omega-3 fatty acids = 1 g, Omega-6 fatty acids = .5 g. Weight Watchers Winning Points = 5

6

Make Your Own Power Bars

At a buck-fifty or more a pop, those tiny power bars can break the bank. And most of these "high performance" bars are missing a friendly dose of ground flaxseed. By making your own power bars you not only save money, but you are able to customize your bars for your own nutritional needs—namely, adding flaxseed. With these tasty recipes (such as Carrot Cake Bars or Lemon Zest Crunch) you will be able to make a batch, wrap them, and freeze them for a totally convenient, compact boost of nutrition that you can take with you anywhere.

Cran-Cherry Oat Bars

MAKES 10 BARS

➳

These bars are a happy medium between a granola bar and a brownie. If you don't care for dried cherries or cranberries, you can substitute any other dried fruit.

4 ounces dried cherries (a slightly heaping ¾ cup measure), finely chopped

4 ounces dried cranberries, like Craisins (a slightly heaping ¾ cup measure), finely chopped

½ cup water

2 teaspoons vanilla extract

1 cup quick cooking oats

½ cup ground flaxseed

1½ cups unbleached or all-purpose flour

¼ cup firmly packed brown sugar

¾ teaspoon baking soda

¾ teaspoon salt

½ cup plus 2 tablespoons light pancake syrup

4 tablespoons butter or canola margarine, melted

⅓ cup finely chopped pecans or walnuts

❖ Combine cherries and cranberries in small saucepan with water and bring to a boil. Reduce heat and simmer until thickened, stirring frequently (about 3 minutes). Remove from heat and stir in vanilla; set aside.

❖ In mixing bowl, combine oats, flaxseed, flour, brown sugar, baking soda, and salt. Mix well with a pastry blender or electric mixer. Drizzle butter and pancake syrup over the top of oat mixture and blend with pastry blender or electric mixer.

❖ Spread 2 cups of oats mixture in the bottom of an 8-inch or 9-inch square baking dish, coated with canola cooking spray, and press firmly. Spread cherry filling evenly on top.

❖ Combine pecans with remaining oat mixture using a pastry blender or fork and pat firmly and evenly on top of filling.

❖ Bake at 350° F in the center of oven for 20 minutes or until golden brown. Let cool.

PER BAR: 303 calories, 5.3 g protein, 47 g carbohydrate, 10 g fat (2.4 g saturated fat, 3.5 g monounsaturated, 2.7 g polyunsaturated fat), 12 mg cholesterol, 5.2 g fiber, 343 mg sodium. Calories from fat: 30 percent. Omega-3 fatty acids = 1.3 g Omega-6 fatty acids = 1.4 g. Weight Watchers Winning Points = 6

Carrot Cake Flax Breakfast Bars

MAKES 10 BARS

ॐ

It may not look like carrot cake, but these moist bars are packed with grated carrot and carrot juice and come complete with a delicious lemon glaze on top.

Canola cooking spray

1½ cups unbleached flour

10 tablespoons ground flaxseed (golden flax works best in this recipe)

½ cup dark brown sugar, packed

1¼ finely grated carrot

2 teaspoons baking powder

1 teaspoon cinnamon

¼ teaspoon salt

1 large egg

½ cup plus 2 tablespoons carrot juice

3 tablespoons canola oil

Lemony Glaze:

½ tablespoon butter or canola margarine, melted

¾ cup powdered sugar

4 teaspoons lemon juice

1½ teaspoons lemon zest, finely chopped

❖ Preheat oven to 350° F. Coat a 9 × 13-inch baking pan with canola cooking spray.

❖ Combine the flour, flaxseed, sugar, carrots, baking powder, cinnamon, and salt in a large mixing bowl; beat on low speed to mix thoroughly.

❖ Add egg, carrot juice, and canola oil to mixing bowl with carrot mixture and beat on low just until blended (be sure not to overbeat).

❖ Spread batter in the prepared pan. Bake until cake is starting to brown and top springs back when gently touched, about 12 minutes.

❖ Combine melted butter, powdered sugar, lemon juice, and lemon zest in small mixing bowl. Blend until smooth. Add a teaspoon or two of extra powdered sugar if necessary for a frosting-like consistency. Spread the top of the bars with the glaze, using the back of a spoon.

PER BAR: 235 calories, 4.5 g protein, 38 g carbohydrate, 8 g fat (1.1 g saturated fat, 3.4 g monounsaturated fat, 3.2 g polyunsaturated fat), 23 mg cholesterol, 3 g fiber, 187 mg sodium. Calories from fat: 31 percent. Omega-3 fatty acids = 1.9 g. Omega-6 fatty acids = 1.3 g. Weight Watchers Winning Points = 5

Cookies & Cream Flax Bars

MAKES 8 GRANOLA BARS

Canola cooking spray

10 reduced-fat chocolate sandwich
cookies, broken into small chunks

1 cup low-fat granola

½ cup ground golden flaxseed (golden
works better in this recipe)

⅓ cup white chocolate chips

½ cup walnut or pecan pieces, coarsely chopped

½ cup fat-free or low-fat sweetened
condensed milk

These decadent bars are for all of you out there who have a sweet tooth and enjoy those cookie-style granola bars.

❖ Preheat oven to 350° F. Coat an 8 × 8-inch baking pan with canola cooking spray.

❖ In a medium-size bowl, combine the cookie chunks, granola, flaxseed, white chocolate chips, and walnuts or pecans, and mix well. Drizzle the condensed milk over the top and stir until well blended.

❖ Using a piece of waxed paper, press the mixture firmly into the prepared pan. Bake for 20 to 25 minutes or until just golden and set. Cool completely.

PER BAR: 239 calories, 5.5 g protein, 40 g carbohydrate, 7 g fat (1.7 g saturated fat, 1.4 g monounsaturated fat, 3.9 g polyunsaturated fat), 3 mg cholesterol, 3.1 g fiber, 109 mg sodium. Calories from fat: 26 percent. Omega-3 fatty acids = 1.5 g, Omega-6 fatty acids = .8 g. Weight Watchers Winning Points = 5

No-Bake Peanut Butter Bars

MAKES 8 BARS

رى

Canola cooking spray

1 tablespoon butter or canola margarine

⅓ cup reduced-fat smooth peanut butter

2 cups miniature marshmallows, lightly packed

1 cup low-fat granola

1 cup Rice Krispies cereal (or other puffed rice cereal)

⅓ cup ground golden flaxseed (golden flax works better in this recipe)

❖ Coat an 8 × 8-inch baking pan with canola cooking spray. Put the butter, peanut butter, and marshmallows into a medium-size microwave-safe bowl and microwave on high for 30 seconds or until the mixture is just melted. Stir to blend.

❖ Microwave again briefly if the mixture isn't melted and smooth. Stir in the granola, puffed rice, and flaxseed.

❖ Spread the mixture in the prepared pan, flattening it evenly with a sheet of waxed paper. Let it cool completely.

PER BAR: 207 calories, 5.5 g protein, 31 g carbohydrate, 8 g fat (2 g saturated fat, 1 g monounsaturated fat, 1.8 g polyunsaturated fat), 4 mg cholesterol, 3 g fiber, 174 mg sodium. Calories from fat: 35 percent. Omega-3 fatty acids = 1 g, Omega-6 fatty acids = .7 g. Weight Watchers Winning Points = 4

Apricot Oat Power Bars

MAKES 10 BARS

❧

1 cup dried apricots, chopped

½ cup sugar

1½ cups water

Canola cooking spray

¾ cup whole wheat flour

¾ cup white flour

1⅓ cups quick or old-fashioned oats

½ cup plus 2 tablespoons ground
   golden flaxseed

½ cup dark brown sugar, packed

1 teaspoon baking soda

1 6-ounce container low-fat or whole
   vanilla or apricot yogurt

3 tablespoons canola oil

¼ cup reduced-calorie pancake syrup,
   regular pancake syrup, or maple
   syrup

1 teaspoon vanilla extract

❖ Add apricots, ½ cup sugar, and 1½ cups water and bring to a boil in small saucepan over medium heat, stirring often. Lower heat and simmer uncovered until fruit thickens to a puree, about 20–25 minutes. Cool completely.

❖ Preheat oven to 350° F. Line a 9 × 9-inch baking dish with foil and coat the foil with canola cooking spray.

❖ Add flour, oats, flaxseed, brown sugar, and baking soda to a large mixing bowl and beat on low to blend. Stir yogurt, canola oil, and vanilla together in 2-cup measure and pour over oat mixture and beat on low, just to blend.

❖ Press half of the oat mixture into pan. Spread with apricot mixture. Crumble remaining oat mixture on top. Gently pat the top into filling. Bake 30 minutes. Store at room temperature in airtight container for up to 1 week.

PER BAR: 320 calories, 6 g protein, 51 g carbohydrate, 10 g fat (1 g saturated fat, 5 g monounsaturated fat, 4 g polyunsaturated fat), 1 mg cholesterol, 4.5 g fiber, 145 mg sodium. Calories from fat: 28 percent. Omega-3 fatty acids = 2.1 g, Omega-6 fatty acids = 1.8 g. Weight Watchers Winning Points = 6

Orange Almond Bars

MAKES 12 BARS

෨

These are not as sweet as other bars, but they still make a tasty treat. They also come in handy when you're pinched for time—if you make a batch and freeze them in a plastic freezer bag, you can just grab one and eat it on the go.

Canola cooking spray

1 cup whole wheat flour

1 cup white all-purpose flour

¾ cup ground golden flax (ground regular flax can also be used)

¼ teaspoon baking soda

¼ cup granulated sugar

½ cup firmly packed brown sugar

¾ cup coarsely chopped blanched almonds (chopped slivered almonds work great)

¼ cup canola oil

¼ cup egg substitute

7 tablespoons fresh (or not from concentrate) orange juice (or similar)

1 tablespoon finely grated orange zest (peel)

1 teaspoon vanilla extract

¾ teaspoon almond extract

❖ Preheat oven to 375° F and coat a 9 × 13-inch baking dish with canola cooking spray.

❖ Add the flours, flaxseed, baking soda, and white and brown sugar, into mixing bowl and beat on low to blend and remove any brown sugar lumps. Stir in almonds.

❖ In a 4-cup measure, whisk the canola oil with the egg substitute, orange juice, orange zest, vanilla, and almond extract until well blended. Pour into the mixing bowl with the dry ingredients and beat on low just until blended.

❖ Pat mixture evenly into prepared pan, using a piece of wax paper to press the mixture down into the pan. Bake until lightly brown and just firm in center, about 13 to 15 minutes.

PER BAR: 240 calories, 6 g protein, 33 g carbohydrate, 9 g fat (1 g saturated, 4 g monounsaturated fat, 4 polyunsaturated fat), 0 mg cholesterol, 5 g fiber, 44 mg sodium. Calories from fat: 35 percent. Omega-3 fatty acids = 2 g, Omega-6 fatty acids = 2 g. Weight Watchers Points = 5

7

Flaxseed Starters

I believe the sky is the limit when it comes to adding flaxseed to our food—even when you're entertaining. I was able to slip some ground flaxseed into a handful of my favorite appetizer recipes, in most cases without anyone being the wiser. These starter dishes are now higher in fiber, pumped up with a little extra phytoestrogens and plant omega-3s, and still absolutely delicious.

Savory Stuffed Mushrooms

ॐ

I know the long list of ingredients may look a bit ominous, but these mushrooms are fairly simple to make and the payoff is worth it—creamy, flavorpacked mushrooms. The flaxseed blends in well because of the sautéed mushrooms stems. If you want to save some time and effort, you can always skip steps #5 and #6 and just bake the mushrooms without the coating.

6 whole baby portobello mushrooms

1 teaspoon canola oil

1½ teaspoons minced garlic

2 teaspoons white wine or nonalcoholic beer

½ cup light cream cheese

3 tablespoons ground flaxseed

3 tablespoons grated Parmesan cheese

2 pinches ground black pepper

2 scallions (green onions), finely chopped (white and part of green)

⅛ teaspoon ground cayenne pepper

¼ cup egg substitute

1½ tablespoons Wondra quick-mixing flour

⅔ cup breadcrumbs (use French bread crumbs if available)

❖ Preheat oven to 450° F. Clean mushrooms with a damp paper towel and carefully break off stems. Finely chop mushrooms stems after cutting off the tough end of the stem; you will have around ⅓ cup.

❖ Heat 1 teaspoon canola oil in medium, nonstick saucepan or frying pan over medium heat. Add garlic, chopped mushroom stems, and wine or beer to skillet. Fry until any moisture has disappeared but be careful not to burn the garlic, about 3 minutes. Turn off heat and let mixture cool about 5 minutes.

❖ Stir cream cheese, flaxseed, Parmesan cheese, black pepper, scallions, and cayenne pepper into mushroom mixture, or blend together using small food processor or electric mixer.

❖ Using a small spoon, fill each mushroom cap well with cream cheese mixture.

❖ Add the egg substitute to a small bowl. Sprinkle Wondra flour over the top and stir with fork until smooth. Add breadcrumbs to another small bowl.

❖ Dip each mushroom, side down, first in egg substitute mixture (dip it only until you come to the top edge of the mushroom—do not dip the filling into the egg) and then in breadcrumbs to coat the outside of the mushroom. Spray outside of mushroom with canola cooking spray. Place mushrooms cap-side down onto prepared baking sheet.

❖ Bake about 30 to 35 minutes or until cream cheese filling is nice and bubbly and mushrooms are cooked throughout.

PER SERVING: 110 calories, 7 g protein, 10 g carbohydrate, 4.7 g fat (1.7 g saturated fat, 1 g monounsaturated fat, 1.2 g polyunsaturated fat), 9 mg cholesterol, 2.3 g fiber, 141 mg sodium. Calories from fat: 38 percent. Omega-3 fatty acids = .8 g Omega-6 fatty acids = .4 g. Weight Watchers Winning Points = 2

Super Easy Sweet and Sour Meatballs

MAKES 6 SERVINGS (ABOUT 10 MEATBALLS EACH)

These meatballs are always the hit of any party I throw. Even though making the meatballs from scratch is a little time-consuming, you save time with the simple sweet and sour sauce.

1 pound super-lean ground beef or ground sirloin

½ cup soft bread crumbs (1–2 slices of bread—whole wheat, sourdough, etc.—finely chopped)

6 tablespoons ground flaxseed

1 egg (¼ cup egg substitute can be substituted)

¼ cup finely minced onion

2 tablespoons low-fat milk or fat-free half-and-half

1½ teaspoons minced or chopped garlic

½ teaspoon salt (optional)

A few dashes of freshly ground pepper

½ cup Heinz chili sauce

½ cup red currant jelly

Canola cooking spray

❖ In a large bowl, combine the first 9 ingredients (everything other than the chili sauce, the jelly, and the cooking spray), mixing well with a wooden spoon or your hands.

❖ Form into about 60 bite-size meatballs.

❖ Start heating a large, nonstick frying pan over medium heat. Coat pan with canola cooking spray and add the meatballs. Lightly brown meatballs, turning them over often. Cover pan and lower heat to simmer and cook an additional 5 minutes or until meatballs are cooked through.

❖ Combine the chili sauce and jelly and pour over the meatballs and simmer gently for about 8 to 10 minutes, stirring and basting the meatballs frequently. Serve with toothpicks if desired.

PER SERVING: 294 calories, 19 g protein, 30 g carbohydrate, 10.5 g fat (3.3 g saturated fat, 3.9 g monounsaturated fat, 2.3 g polyunsaturated fat), 63 mg cholesterol, 3 g fiber, 738 mg sodium. Calories from fat: 32 percent. Omega-3 fatty acids = 1.5 g Omega-6 fatty acids = .5 g. Weight Watchers Winning Points = 6

Spiral Spinach Bacon Bites

MAKES 8 APPETIZER SERVINGS (6 BITES EACH) OR 4 WRAP SANDWICHES

౭

Eat these appetizers cold or serve them hot from the oven—either way they're delicious. You can also fashion them into tasty wrap sandwiches if you prefer.

1 10-ounce package frozen chopped spinach, thawed and gently squeezed of excess water

¼ cup ground flaxseed (golden flax works best in this recipe)

4 ounces light cream cheese

1 tablespoon real mayonnaise (or canola mayonnaise)

3 tablespoons fat-free or light sour cream

½ teaspoon salt (optional)

½ teaspoon pepper

½ cup chopped green onions (about 3)

6 strips Louis Rich turkey bacon, cooked until crisp and crumbled into small pieces

4 7-inch flour tortillas (or use 3 of the 9-inch size)

Canola cooking spray

PER SERVING: 174 calories, 7.5 g protein, 18.5 g carbohydrate, 8 g fat (2 g saturated fat, 2.4 g monounsaturated fat, 2.5 g polyunsaturated fat), 15 mg cholesterol, 3.2 g fiber, 350 mg sodium. Calories from fat: 40 percent. Omega-3 fatty acids = .8 g Omega-6 fatty acids = .9 g. Weight Watchers Winning Points = 3

❖ Combine the first seven ingredients in mixing bowl and blend with a mixer on low speed until thoroughly blended.

❖ Add green onions and bacon bits and beat on low until mixed in.

❖ Lay a large square of plastic wrap on flat surface. Lay a soft tortilla on top. Spread ¼ of filling evenly on the tortilla using a scraper. Roll up tortilla tightly, enclosing the filling. Wrap the plastic tightly around it.

❖ Repeat with remaining tortillas and filling. Chill rolls until filling is firm (at least 1 hour or up to 24 hours).

❖ Remove plastic and if you are serving them as appetizers, cut rolls crosswise on slight diagonal into ¾-inch thick slices. Serve cold or if you prefer them heated, preheat oven to 400°F. Arrange slices on a large baking sheet lined with foil then coated with canola cooking spray. Bake until heated through, about 7 minutes. You can also eat these as wrap sandwiches.

Florentine Artichoke Dip

MAKES 8 SMALL APPETIZER SERVINGS
OR 4 LARGE APPETIZER SERVINGS

This tastes similar to the famous hot artichoke dip, but it has some added antioxidants and fiber from chopped spinach and the flaxseed and a lot less fat.

Canola cooking spray

1 8-ounce package light cream cheese

1 tablespoon real mayonnaise (or
canola mayonnaise)

3 tablespoons fat-free or light sour
cream

6½ ounce jar marinated or water-
packed artichoke hearts, drained
and chopped

1 10-ounce box frozen chopped
spinach, thawed and gently
squeezed of excess water

½ cup shredded Parmesan cheese

1½ teaspoons minced garlic

1½ tablespoons lemon juice

¼ teaspoon Tabasco

¼ cup ground golden flaxseed (golden
flax hides better in this recipe)

freshly ground pepper to taste (about
⅛ teaspoon)

❖ Preheat oven to 375° F. Coat an 8-inch quiche dish (an 8- or 9-inch pie plate can also be used) with canola cooking spray; set aside.

❖ In medium mixing bowl, blend together the cream cheese, mayonnaise, and sour cream on low speed until smooth. Beat in the artichoke hearts, spinach, Parmesan cheese, garlic, lemon juice, Tabasco, and flaxseed.

❖ Spread evenly into the prepared dish and sprinkle freshly ground pepper over the top. Bake uncovered for 20 to 25 minutes or until the surface is lightly browned and bubbly. Serve with bread and crackers of your choice.

SERVING SUGGESTIONS: Serve with sliced baguette, reduced fat Triscuits or Wheat Thins, or any reduced fat cracker that you enjoy.

PER SMALL APPETIZER SERVING: (not including bread or crackers): 118 calories, 8 g protein, 7 g carbohydrate, 6.5 g fat (2.8 g saturated fat, 1.1 g monounsaturated fat, 1.8 g polyunsaturated fat), 15 mg cholesterol, 3 g fiber, 343 mg sodium. Calories from fat: 49 percent. Omega-3 fatty acids = .8 g, Omega-6 fatty acids = .2 g. Weight Watchers Winning Points = 2

NOTE: If you want to know what a larger appetizer serving would contain, just double the nutritional analysis information.

Seven-Layer Mexican Bean Dip

MAKES 6 HEARTY OR 12 SMALL APPETIZER SERVINGS

જી

This is easier to fix than it looks and it goes over real well at a casual party or barbeque—even the kids love it.

1 16-ounce can fat-free or vegetarian refried beans (or similar)

⅓ cup ground flaxseed (golden will work best in this recipe)

½ to 1 teaspoon chili powder (depending on how spicy you like it)

Black pepper to taste

½ teaspoon pepper sauce to taste, green or red, mild or hot (like Tobasco)

¾ cup plus 1 tablespoon fat-free or light sour cream

1 avocado, mashed

1½ teaspoons lemon juice

¾ cup grated reduced-fat sharp cheddar cheese

1 cup finely chopped tomatoes

5 green onions, chopped

2 ounces chopped black olives (optional)

❖ Heat beans in small nonstick saucepan over low heat until warm and softened. Stir in flaxseed, chili powder, black pepper, and pepper sauce to taste. Spread into 8 × 8-inch baking dish (or similar) and let cool.

❖ Spread sour cream over the beans.

❖ In small bowl or small food processor, blend avocado with the tablespoon sour cream and 1½ teaspoons lemon juice. Spread this guacamole mixture evenly over the sour cream layer.

❖ Sprinkle grated cheese over the avocado layer, then top the cheese evenly with chopped tomatoes.

❖ Sprinkle green onions and then olives (if desired) over the tomatoes. Cover dish and refrigerate until needed.

SUGGESTED DIPPERS: Reduced-fat or regular tortilla chips, soft flour tortillas, or pita bread cut into triangles

PER SMALL APPETIZER SERVING (JUST THE DIP): 120 calories, 6 g protein, 12 g carbohydrate, 5.5 g fat (1.6 g saturated fat, 1.7 g monounsaturated fat, 1.5 g polyunsaturated fat), 6 mg cholesterol, 4 g fiber, 240 mg sodium. Calories from fat: 41 percent. Omega-3 fatty acids = .7 g, Omega-6 fatty acids = .5 gram. Weight Watchers Winning Points = 2

Light Wild Mushroom Paté

You can make this a day or two ahead of a party or special occasion. Although several types of mushrooms can be used, I used portobello, which works great.

½ cup walnuts, finely chopped (plus more for garnish if desired)

1½ tablespoons butter

1 pound assorted mushrooms, such as portabella, crimini, shiitake, and white button, cleaned and coarsely chopped (about 6 cups)

6 green onions, white and part green, finely chopped

1 tablespoon fresh thyme leaves, finely chopped (plus more for garnish, if desired)

¾ teaspoon salt

½ teaspoon freshly ground black pepper

¼ cup dry sherry

Juice from ½ lemon

½ cup fresh flat-leaf parsley leaves, finely chopped

2–3 dashes Tabasco sauce

½ cup light cream cheese

¼ cup ground flaxseed

❖ Heat oven to 350° F. Spread walnuts on a baking pan and bake until fragrant, about 7 minutes. Transfer walnuts to a bowl and set aside to cool.

❖ In a large, nonstick skillet over medium heat, melt butter and cook the chopped mushrooms and green onions, stirring occasionally, until liquid has been released and the skillet becomes almost dry, about 10 minutes. Stir in thyme, salt, and pepper. Cook 2 more minutes. Add sherry and cook until skillet is almost dry, about 4 minutes. Stir in lemon juice and remove from heat to cool.

❖ In mixing bowl, combine the mushroom mixture, toasted walnuts, fresh parsley, Tabasco sauce, cream cheese, and flaxseed together, beating on low speed. Add more salt and pepper to taste if desired.

❖ Line a 3-cup mold (a 9-inch loaf pan will also do fine) with plastic wrap, allowing for a 4-inch overhang on all sides. Spoon the mushroom mixture into the prepared mold or pan. Firmly press down all over the mold with your hands, spreading mixture as evenly as possible. Cover the mold with the overhanging plastic and chill in the refrigerator for at least 8 hours or overnight.

❖ Just before serving, unwrap the mold or loaf pan and invert it onto the serving plate. Garnish with extra walnuts and thyme leaves if desired. Serve with toast-points (made from thin-sliced sandwich bread: remove crusts, and toast until just golden) or crackers.

PER SERVING: (NOT INCLUDING BREAD OR CRACKERS) 95 calories, 4 g protein, 4.5 g carbohydrate, 6.5 g fat (2 g saturated fat, 1.1 g monounsaturated fat, 2.7 g polyunsaturated fat), 9 mg cholesterol, 2.5 g fiber, 249 mg sodium. Calories from fat: 62 percent. Omega-3 fatty acids = 1 gram Omega-6 fatty acids = 1.7 g. Weight Watchers Winning Points = 2

Sun-Dried Tomato Pesto Torta

MAKES 6 APPETIZER SERVINGS

You can buy these pre-made in the supermarket, but they are going to have a lot more fat grams and calories and they won't have our featured ingredient—flaxseed. This comes out looking so beautiful, with its green and red layers, perfect for the holiday season.

8 ounces light cream cheese, divided in half (fat-free cream cheese can be substituted and will reduce the fat grams by about 5 grams per serving)

⅓ cup store-bought pesto (I like Armanino pesto in the frozen section)

½ cup well-drained, oil-packed sun-dried tomatoes, finely chopped

2½ tablespoons tomato paste

¼ cup ground golden flaxseed (golden works best in this recipe)

⅛ cup toasted pine nuts (optional)

SERVING SUGGESTIONS: Serve with water crackers, reduced-fat wheat crackers, or baguette slices.

PER SERVING (NOT INCLUDING BREAD OR CRACKERS): 190 calories, 9 g protein, 10 g carbohydrate, 12.5 g fat (3.7 g saturated fat, 5 g monounsaturated fat, 3.5 g polyunsaturated fat), 17 mg cholesterol, 3.1 g fiber, 398 mg sodium. Calories from fat: 62 percent. Omega-3 fatty acids = 1 gram Omega-6 fatty acids = 1.5 g. Weight Watchers Winning Points = 4

❖ Add 4 ounces of light cream cheese and ½ cup of pesto to small mixing bowl. Beat on low speed until blended very well.

❖ Add sun-dried tomatoes, tomato paste, remaining 4 ounces of light cream cheese, and flaxseed to small food processor and pulse until mixture is well blended.

❖ Line a 2 to 3-cup soufflé dish (or similar) with plastic wrap—enough so plenty is hanging over the sides. Spread half of the pesto mixture evenly in the bottom of the prepared dish. Top with half of the sun-dried tomato mixture, then the remaining pesto mixture. Then spread the remaining sun-dried tomato mixture evenly on top of the final pesto layer. Cover the torta well with the plastic wrap hanging outside the soufflé dish. Chill in refrigerator overnight (can be made 2 days ahead).

❖ When ready to serve, unwrap the top of the torta, then invert onto a serving platter. Peel off plastic completely. Garnish the top with basil sprigs and toasted pine nuts, if desired. Serve with baguette slices and/or crackers.

8

Awesome Entrées

In this section, you'll find some of our most revered American comfort foods transformed into new and quick flaxseed-fortified—and often lower-fat—recipes. You are probably thinking, I can see adding flaxseed to a smoothie or a loaf of bread, but an entrée? Hey, when you are trying to add a tablespoon or two of ground flaxseed to your diet each day, 365 days a year, you need lots of options. You can't have a smoothie every day. And you probably don't have the time to mix up a batch of muffins or bake some bread every few days either. Enter the entrée.

You will be surprised how easy it is to stir a tablespoon of flaxseed into certain entrées—I know I was pleasantly surprised—and you'll find that certain dishes lend themselves to hiding flax. Entrées with dark red sauces, like chili, sloppy joes, spaghetti, or minestrone work well, along with rolled-up or mixed-up and molded dishes, like enchiladas, flautas, meatloaf, and stuffed peppers.

I have to admit that this became my favorite way to work my token tablespoon of flax into my day.

This chapter is filled with flaxseed remakes of beloved meat and casserole–type recipes—recipes most of us love to make and eat over and over. Whenever possible, the following recipes have been trimmed of any excess fat and calories; olive oil and canola oil are the chosen fat; and time-saving tricks have been employed.

Ham and Swiss Frittata with Asparagus

MAKES 2 SERVINGS (OR SERVES 4 AS A SIDE DISH OR APPETIZER)

ॐ

Frittatas are the ultimate one-pan meal. I usually try to decoratively arrange asparagus spears or tomato half-slices over the top of the frittata, for color and a little added nutrition.

½ cup finely chopped onion

½ cup finely chopped green bell pepper

Salt and pepper to taste

2 teaspoons olive oil

2 large eggs

½ cup egg substitute

½ cup chopped cooked lean ham
  (about 3 ounces)

½ cup grated reduced-fat Swiss or
  Jarlsberg cheese (about 2 ounces)

2 tablespoons ground flaxseed

canola or olive oil cooking spray

8 asparagus spears, lightly cooked, or
  1 vine-ripened tomato, cut into
  half-circle slices

½ teaspoon Italian seasoning (or any
  herb blend you like)

PER SERVING (½ FRITTATA):
336 calories, 32 g protein, 18 g carbohydrate, 15 g fat (6.5 g saturated fat, 3.3 g mono-unsaturated fat, 2.8 g polyunsaturated fat), 242 mg cholesterol, 6 g fiber, 743 mg sodium. Calories from fat: 40 percent. Omega-3 fatty acids = 1.5 g, Omega-6 fatty acids = 1.2 g. Weight Watchers Winning Points = 7

❖ In a 9-inch, nonstick skillet, cook the onion and bell pepper with salt and pepper to taste in 2 teaspoons oil over medium heat, stirring often, until the bell pepper is tender, about 3 minutes.

❖ In a mixing bowl, beat or whisk together the eggs, egg substitute, ham, and Swiss cheese. Add the bell pepper mixture and flaxseed and beat or whisk until well combined.

❖ Start heating the 9-inch skillet again over medium heat until hot. Coat the pan generously with canola cooking spray and quickly pour in the egg mixture, distributing the ham and bell peppers evenly. While it begins to cook, arrange asparagus spears or tomato slices decoratively on top, then sprinkle ½ teaspoon of Italian seasoning on top. Cover the skillet and cook (without stirring) for about 6 minutes, or until the frittata is set and bottom is nicely brown.

❖ If desired, broil the frittata under a preheated broiler, about 4 inches from the heat, for 2 minutes—to lightly brown the top. Let cool in the skillet for 5 minutes. Slide the frittata onto a serving plate, cut into wedges, and serve it warm or at room temperature.

Spinach Quiche Lorraine

چو

This recipe is very easy to make, especially if you use one of those ready-made piecrusts. Just mix up the filling ingredients, dump it in, and bake!

1 10-inch pie crust (such as Pillsbury ready-made)

8 slices Louis Rich turkey bacon, cooked and crumbled

1 cup Jarlsberg Lite or reduced-fat Swiss cheese, firmly packed

1 9-ounce box frozen chopped spinach (thawed, extra water gently squeezed out)

½ cup ground flaxseed

½ cup chopped green onions

3 tablespoons Wondra quick-mixing flour

⅛ cup mayonnaise

¾ cup fat-free sour cream

2 large eggs

½ cup egg substitute

1 cup low-fat milk

¼ teaspoon ground pepper (optional)

½ teaspoon garlic powder, and dried oregano leaves (optional)

❖ Preheat oven to 375° F. Lay pie crust in deep-dish pie dish.

❖ Add bacon, cheese, spinach, flaxseed, and green onions to medium bowl and toss to blend. Spread into crust-lined pie dish.

❖ Add flour, mayonnaise, and sour cream to mixing bowl and beat on low to blend well. Scrape sides of bowl with spoon. While on low speed, add eggs, one at a time, then egg substitute, ¼ cup at a time.

❖ Slowly beat in milk until mixture is blended and smooth. Beat in pepper or garlic and oregano if desired. Pour into pie dish. Bake for about 40 minutes or until a knife inserted into the center comes out clean.

PER SERVING (WITH CRUST): 319 calories, 16 g protein, 21 g carbohydrate, 19 g fat (6 g saturated fat, 6.4 g monounsaturated fat, 5 g polyunsaturated fat), 80 mg cholesterol, 4 g fiber, 493 mg sodium. Calories from fat: 54 percent. Omega-3 fatty acids = 1.6 g Omega-6 fatty acids = 1.9 g. Weight Watchers Winning Points = 7

Pesto Pasta Salad

MAKES 10 SERVINGS

༂

This is one of my favorite pasta recipes—the colors are beautiful and the flavors blend perfectly. Best of all, it is easy to make. And when you use golden flaxseed in this recipe, it almost looks like there are ground pine nuts in the pesto sauce.

12 ounces pasta noodles of choice, dried (rotelle, penne, etc.)

⅓ cup pine nuts

1 cup fresh basil, rinsed and well drained

2 cups chopped vine-ripened tomatoes or quartered cherry tomatoes

2 jars (6 ounces each) artichoke hearts (water packed or marinated), rinsed and drained

1 7-ounce container Armanino pesto sauce (in frozen food section of your supermarket) *or* 14 tablespoons of another pesto made with olive oil or canola oil, thawed

¼ cup ground golden flaxseed (golden flax works better in this recipe)

3 tablespoons grated Parmesan cheese

❖ Start boiling water in large saucepan. When water is boiling, add noodles and continue to boil until pasta is tender (according to directions on package), about 10 to 12 minutes, then drain well in collander.

❖ While noodles are boiling, toast pine nuts in 400° F oven (use 300° F if using a toaster oven) until light brown, watching carefully (about 3 to 5 minutes). Cool and add to serving bowl.

❖ Coarsely chop fresh basil; add to serving bowl. Chop tomatoes and artichoke hearts and add to serving bowl.

❖ In small bowl, combine pesto sauce with flaxseed. Add drained noodles to serving bowl along with pesto-flaxseed mixture and Parmesan cheese and toss everything together well. Store in refrigerator until needed.

PER SERVING: 260 calories, 10 g protein, 34 g carbohydrate, 10 g fat (2 g saturated fat, 4.4 g monounsaturated fat, 3.5 g polyunsaturated fat), 5 mg cholesterol, 5 g fiber, 365 mg sodium. Calories from fat: 37 percent. Omega-3 fatty acids = .8 gram Omega-6 fatty acids = 1 gram. Weight Watchers Winning Points = 5

Crab Cakes with Quick Jalapeño-Lime Mayonnaise

MAKES 6 ENTRÉE SERVINGS (12 APPETIZER SERVINGS)

و

If the price of crabmeat makes this recipe prohibitive, you can use imitation crabmeat, but you'll need to shred it into smaller pieces so it will blend better with the rest of the ingredients. Another way to go is to buy half of a pound of real crabmeat and half of a pound of imitation.

2 tablespoons canola oil, divided

1 cup finely diced white onions

1 cup finely diced celery

1 pound fresh crabmeat

¼ cup egg substitute (1 lightly beaten egg can be substituted)

1½ tablespoons Dijon mustard

1–2 tablespoons finely chopped fresh parsley (or 1½ teaspoons dried)

1 tablespoon finely chopped fresh thyme (or 1 teaspoon dried)

Salt and pepper to taste

Cayenne pepper to taste (optional)

1⅔ cup fine white bread crumbs (sourdough or French if available), divided

⅓ cup ground flaxseed

Canola cooking spray

Jalapeño-Lime Mayonnaise:

2 tablespoons real mayonnaise

½ cup fat-free sour cream (light can also be used)

2 tablespoons lime juice

1 teaspoon seeded and minced jalapeño pepper (add more to taste)

½ teaspoon Dijon mustard

Salt, pepper, and cayenne pepper to taste

❖ Heat 1 tablespoon of the oil in a large nonstick skillet or frying pan, and cook onion and celery over medium heat until tender, about 4 minutes. Place mixture in a small food processor and pulse a few times to make mixture finer, or use a food chopper or knife.

❖ Place crabmeat, onion mixture, egg substitute, and mustard in mixing bowl and blend on low speed. Add parsley, thyme, salt, pepper, cayenne (if desired), and ⅔ cup of bread crumbs and ground flaxseed to crabmeat mixture and beat on low speed just until blended.

❖ Form crab mixture into 12 small cakes. Use a ⅓-cup measure to help shape the mixture, then pat it into ½-inch-thick cakes. Roll the crab cakes into the remaining 1 cup of bread crumbs.

❖ Heat remaining tablespoon of canola oil in the same skillet or frying pan over medium heat. Lightly brown crab cakes on each side, 2 to 3 minutes, turning once (coat pan or top of crab cakes with canola cooking spray as needed). Serve with Jalapeño-Lime Mayonnaise as dipping sauce.

❖ For mayonnaise: Combine mayonnaise, sour cream, lime juice, jalapeño, and mustard in a food processor or 2-cup measure. Blend until smooth. Adjust seasoning and minced jalapeño to taste.

PER ENTRÉE SERVING (INCLUDING JALAPEÑO-LIME MAYO): 244 calories, 20 g protein, 13 g carbohydrate, 12 g fat (1.5 g saturated fat, 5 g monounsaturated fat, 5.5 g polyunsaturated fat), 44 mg cholesterol, 3 g fiber, 999 mg sodium. Calories from fat: 44 percent. Omega-3 fatty acids 2.1 g, Omega-6 fatty acids 1.4 g. Weight Watchers Winning Points = 5

Chicken Fettuccini Alfredo

MAKES 4 TO 6 SERVINGS

ↄ

Creamy and spicy—a combination made in heaven. But if you don't think your children will like the chicken strips seasoned with spicy Old Bay Seasoning, just sprinkle it on half the chicken strips.

4 chicken breasts (half breasts), skinless and boneless

Canola cooking spray

¼–½ teaspoon Old Bay Seasoning (half of the chicken strips can be seasoned with salt, pepper, and garlic powder instead of Old Bay, if desired)

¼ cup light cream cheese

1 cup whole milk, divided use

1 tablespoon Wondra quick-mixing flour

1½ tablespoons butter (canola margarine can also be used)

6 cups hot cooked and drained spaghetti or fettuccini noodles

Salt and freshly grated pepper to taste

Nutmeg to taste

⅓ cup shredded Parmesan cheese (add more at table if desired)

4 tablespoons ground golden flaxseed (golden flax works best in this recipe)

❖ Start boiling fettuccini noodles now if you haven't already done so.

❖ Cut each chicken breast into about 6 thin strips, cutting lengthwise to make the longest strips possible.

❖ Start heating a large nonstick frying pan or skillet over medium-high heat. When hot, coat with canola cooking spray. Add the chicken strips immediately. Spray the tops with canola cooking spray then sprinkle with Old Bay Seasoning and let brown for about 3 to 4 minutes. Flip strips around and brown other side (about 3 to 4 minutes). Test the thickest strip to check that it is cooked through, then cover pan and turn off heat.

❖ Combine cream cheese, ¼ cup whole milk, and flour in a small mixing bowl or food processor. Beat or pulse until well blended. Slowly pour in remaining milk (¾ cup) and beat until smooth.

❖ Melt butter in large, nonstick frying pan or saucepan over medium heat. Add the milk mixture and continue to heat, stirring constantly, until the sauce is just the right thickness, about 4 minutes.

❖ Turn the heat to low and add the hot noodles and chicken strips. Toss to generously coat noodles and chicken with sauce. Add salt, pepper, and nutmeg to taste if desired. Stir in grated Parmesan and golden flax (add ½ tablespoon to 1 tablespoon of golden flax per serving—depending on your taste and motivation). Serve hot.

PER SERVING (IF 6 SERVINGS): 400 calories, 30 g protein, 48 g carbohydrate, 10.5 g fat (5 g saturated fat, 2.4 g monounsaturated fat, 2 g polyunsaturated fat), 66 mg cholesterol, 4 g fiber, 227 mg sodium. Calories from fat: 24 percent. Omega-3 fatty acids = 1.7 g Omega-6 fatty acids = 1.3 g. Weight Watchers Winning Points = 7

Pizza Sticks

ॐ

These are a blast both to make and to eat! I use frozen bread dough, string cheese, and bottled pizza sauce, which makes them even simpler to do.

1 48-ounce package of White Bridgeford Ready-Dough (in frozen food section of most supermarkets), thawed in refrigerator

18 string cheeses (low moisture part-skim mozzarella in sticks)

Garlic powder to sprinkle (about 1 tablespoon altogether)

Salt to sprinkle, about 1 teaspoon altogether (optional)

Italian herb seasoning to sprinkle (about 1 tablespoon altogether)

Ground golden flaxseed to sprinkle, about ½ cup altogether (golden flax will work best in this recipe)

Canola cooking spray

1½ tablespoons butter, melted (or olive oil)

⅛ cup shredded Parmesan cheese

Bottled pizza sauce

❖ Cut each 1-pound loaf of dough into 6 equal portions (the ball of dough will fill about a ½-cup measure).

❖ Lay a large piece of wax paper on a flat surface and lightly sprinkle with flour.

❖ Place a ball of dough on the wax paper and press it into a rectangle about 6 inches long and 3 inches wide.

❖ On the top of the dough sprinkle some garlic powder (about ⅛ teaspoon) and a little salt (if desired), some Italian herb seasoning (about ⅛ teaspoon), and some ground flaxseed (about 1½ teaspoons). While holding the dough in its 6 × 3-inch shape, place one of the string cheese sticks down the center and roll the dough around it, sealing the edges of the dough together by crimping them with your fingers. Place the pizza sticks 2 inches apart on jellyroll pans or baking sheets that have been coated with canola cooking spray.

❖ Repeat Steps 3 and 4 with the rest of the dough, cheese sticks, and seasonings, dusting the wax paper with flour as needed.

❖ When all the pizza sticks are in the prepared pans, brush the top of each stick generously with melted butter or olive oil. Then sprinkle the top of each stick with some Parmesan cheese.

❖ Preheat oven to 400° F while you let the pizza sticks rest and rise for about 20 minutes. Bake until nicely brown on top and the dough is no longer raw, about 18 minutes.

❖ Serve sticks with bottled pizza sauce for dipping!

PER STICK: 301 calories, 16.5 g protein, 43 g carbohydrate, 7 g fat (4.8 g saturated fat, .6 g monounsaturated fat, .9 g polyunsaturated fat), 23 mg cholesterol, 4 g fiber, 832 mg sodium (sodium might be lower if you use a lower sodium pizza or marinara sauce). Calories from fat: 27 percent. Omega-3 fatty acids = .7 g Omega-6 fatty acids = .2. Weight Watchers Winning Points = 6

Artichoke Torte

MAKES 9 SERVINGS

࿊

I work at home so I am always looking for foods I can have in the fridge or freezer that are only a two-minute microwave setting away from becoming a warm, ready-to-eat meal. I make this one all the time.

Canola cooking spray

4 large eggs

1 cup egg substitute

3 tablespoons pesto (I use the Armanino brand in the frozen food section)

1 teaspoon garlic powder

2 teaspoons Italian herb seasoning

⅔ cup plain breadcrumbs

⅓ cup ground flaxseed (golden flax works best with this recipe)

½ cup finely chopped white or yellow onion

1 cup shredded Parmesan cheese

2 cans (13¾ ounces each) quartered artichoke hearts, drained well

2 tomatoes, sliced

❖ Preheat oven to 400° F. Coat a 9 × 9-inch or 8 × 8-inch baking dish with canola cooking spray.

❖ In large mixing bowl, beat the eggs and egg substitute together on medium speed. Beat in the pesto, garlic powder, and Italian herb seasoning.

❖ Reduce the speed to low and add the breadcrumbs, flaxseed, onion, and Parmesan cheese.

❖ Stir in the drained artichoke hearts and pour into prepared dish. Level the top by spreading with a spatula or scraper. Press tomato slices gently all over the top.

❖ Bake until lightly brown on the outside, about 45 minutes.

PER SERVING: 189 calories, 14 g protein, 16.5 g carbohydrate, 7.5 g fat (2.7 g saturated fat, 2.5 g monounsaturated fat, 2 g polyunsaturated fat), 102 mg cholesterol, 5 g fiber, 750 mg sodium. Calories from fat: 36 percent. Omega-3 fatty acids = .9 gram Omega-6 fatty acids = .6 gram. Weight Watchers Winning Points = 3

Ten-Minute Spaghetti Carbonara—
The No-Egg-Yolk Version

MAKES 2 TO 4 SERVINGS (2 LARGE SERVINGS OR 4 SMALL SERVINGS)

کٮ

This is really easy to make, especially if you use leftover spaghetti noodles. I consider this the perfect recipe for one of those busy back-to-school week-nights.

4 cups cooked spaghetti noodles
  (cooked until tender but still a little
  firm), drained

¼ cup egg substitute

1 tablespoon Wondra quick-mixing
  flour

½ cup plus 2 tablespoons double-
  strength chicken broth

¼ cup dry white wine (champagne
  may also be used)

2 garlic cloves, minced (about 2 teaspoons)

1½ tablespoons butter

⅛ cup ground golden flaxseed (golden
  flax works best in this recipe)

Salt and freshly ground pepper
  (optional)

4 slices Louis Rich turkey bacon,
  cooked carefully over medium-low
  heat and crumbled

½ cup freshly grated Parmesan cheese
  (add more to taste if desired)

❖ Boil spaghetti noodles if you haven't already done so. In a small bowl, blend egg substitute with the Wondra flour; set aside.

❖ In large nonstick skillet, combine the chicken broth, wine, garlic, and butter. Bring the mixture to a boil. Let boil gently for a minute or two. Turn off the heat and stir in the flaxseed. Season mixture with salt and pepper, if desired.

❖ Turn off heat. Add in the egg substitute mixture, stir well. Add the warm spaghetti noodles and toss well.

❖ Stir in the crumbled turkey bacon and Parmesan cheese and toss well.

PER SERVING (IF 4 SERVINGS): 368 calories, 18 g protein, 43 g carbohydrate, 13 g fat (5.6 g saturated fat, 3.9 g monounsaturated fat, 2.5 g polyunsaturated fat), 31 mg cholesterol, 3.5 g fiber, 671 mg sodium. Calories from fat: 31 percent. Omega-3 fatty acids = .9 gram Omega-6 fatty acids = 1.6 g. Weight Watchers Winning Points = 8

Green Eggs, Ham, and Spinach Benedict

MAKES 4 SERVINGS

✥

For this recipe, you'll end up with more hollandaise sauce than you'll know what to do with. If you refrigerate the remaining sauce in a covered container, it will keep for several days—just reheat in microwave.

4 large eggs (use high–omega-3 eggs if available in your supermarket)

8 small circular slices of lean ham (8 slices of Canadian bacon can also be used)

Canola cooking spray

Light Hollandaise Sauce:

   3 large egg yolks

   6 tablespoons egg substitute

   4 tablespoons lemon juice (to taste)

   2 tablespoons butter

   ⅓ cup fat-free or light sour cream

   1 tablespoon cornstarch

   ⅓ cup low-fat milk

   Salt and pepper to taste (about ½ teaspoon salt and a couple pinches pepper)

4 English muffins

1 cup frozen chopped spinach, thawed and lightly squeezed of excess water (about half of an 11-ounce box)

¼ cup ground flaxseed

❖ Poach 4 eggs in pot boiling water, place on plate, cover with foil, and set aside.

❖ Pan-fry 8 circles of ham in nonstick skillet coated with canola cooking spray until nicely browned; set aside.

❖ Place the 3 egg yolks, 6 tablespoons egg substitute, and 4 tablespoons lemon juice in an 8-cup glass measuring bowl (a medium glass bowl would work). Beat with a wire whisk until smooth. Place in microwave and heat on HIGH for 1 minute.

❖ Stir with whisk and heat again for 1 minute or until the egg mixture is noticeably hot. Add butter and stir until butter is completely melted.

❖ Blend ⅓ cup sour cream with cornstarch, then slowly whisk in the ⅓ cup milk—blend until smooth. Whisk sour cream mixture into the egg yolk mixture—blend until smooth.

❖ Microwave on high for about 3 or 4 minutes, whisking after each minute, until hollandaise sauce is desired thickness. Add salt and pepper to taste.

❖ Split English muffins and toast each until lightly browned. Add a circle of ham to each half. Blend spinach with ground flaxseed in small bowl. Top each English muffin half with about ⅛ cup of spinach mixture. Set the two English muffin halves side by side on each plate and top both halves with one of the poached eggs. Top each egg with about ¼ cup of hollandaise sauce. Microwave on high about 2 minutes to heat through and serve.

PER SERVING: 385 calories, 25 g protein, 35.5 g carbohydrate, 16 g fat (5.2 g saturated fat, 5.2 g monounsaturated fat, 3.6 g polyunsaturated fat), 321 mg cholesterol, 5 g fiber, 1,031 mg sodium. Calories from fat: 37 percent. Omega-3 fatty acids = 1.7 g Omega-6 fatty acids = 1.9 g. Weight Watchers Winning Points = 8

Old-Fashioned Stovetop Beef Stew

MAKES 6 SERVINGS

There's nothing like the smell of beef stew simmering on the stovetop on a cold winter day. Of course it doesn't hurt that this recipe hides the flaxseed really well, too.

½ cup unbleached flour (or all-purpose)

1 tablespoon garlic powder

1 teaspoon salt (add more to taste if desired)

½ teaspoon black pepper (add more to taste if desired)

1 pound beef stew meat (cut into 3/4-inch cubes)

1 tablespoon canola oil

Canola cooking spray

½ cup coarsely chopped onions

3 medium potatoes, diced

2 cups baby carrots

2 large stalks celery, sliced

2 cups beef broth

1 14.5-ounce can Italian-style diced tomatoes, including juice

1 teaspoon oregano flakes

6 tablespoons ground flaxseed

PER SERVING: 374 calories, 24 g protein, 43 g carbohydrate, 11.5 g fat (3 g saturated fat, 4.8 g monounsaturated fat, 2.8 g polyunsaturated fat), 58 mg cholesterol, 8 g fiber, 1147 mg sodium. Calories from fat: 28 percent. Omega-3 fatty acids = 1.7 g Omega-6 fatty acids = 1.1 g. Weight Watchers Winning Points = 7

❖ Add flour, garlic powder, salt, and pepper to a medium-sized bowl and blend well. Add a handful of the beef cubes to the flour and toss to coat well; set coated cubes aside on a plate. Repeat until all the beef cubes are coated with the flour mixture.

❖ In large, nonstick saucepan over medium-high heat, begin heating the tablespoons of oil. Spread bottom of pan with the oil, then add the beef cubes. Spray the tops with canola cooking spray. Brown the meat, turning the cubes often to brown all sides.

❖ Lower heat to medium and add chopped onions and continue to stir and brown onions for 2 minutes more.

❖ Add diced potatoes, baby carrots, sliced celery, beef broth, diced tomatoes, juice, and oregano to saucepan and stir everything together well. Bring stew to a boil. Reduce heat to low, cover, and simmer for 2 hours, stirring occasionally. The stew is ready to eat when beef is tender and cooked through along with the carrots and potatoes. Stir in 6 tablespoons of ground flaxseed and spoon into 6 serving bowls.

Ham and Hash Brown Casserole

MAKES 12 SERVINGS

ॐ

This is a delicious meal even without the ham. If you don't have ham or want to make this as a side dish, just delete the ham and call it Hash Brown Casserole. The original recipe calls for adding ½ cup melted butter and a container of sour cream. I use 2 tablespoons butter plus 6 tablespoons chicken broth, and fat-free or light sour cream instead. To top this casserole, some versions of the recipe call for crumbled potato chips; others call for sautéeing crushed cornflakes in half a stick of butter. I opt for the cornflakes and coated them with canola cooking spray instead of sautéeing them in butter.

Canola cooking spray

1 14-ounce package frozen country-style hash brown potatoes, thawed

2 tablespoons melted butter

6 tablespoons chicken broth

1 10¾-ounce can condensed cream of chicken soup

8 ounces fat-free or light sour cream

1 cup chopped onions

1½ cups shredded, reduced-fat sharp cheddar cheese

2 cups extra lean ham, cubed or chopped

½ cup ground flaxseed (golden flax will hide better in this recipe)

1 teaspoon salt (optional)

¼ teaspoon ground black pepper

2 cups crushed golden flax cereal (cornflakes can also be used . . . or any other ground flaxseed containing flake cereal. Just use your hands to crush the flakes into a 2-cup measure)

❖ Preheat oven to 350° F. Coat a $9 \times 13 \times 2$-inch baking dish with canola cooking spray.

❖ Add hash browns, butter, broth, condensed cream of chicken soup, sour cream, chopped onion, cheese, ham, flaxseed, salt (if desired), and pepper to a large bowl and stir to blend well. Place mixture in prepared baking dish.

❖ Sprinkle flax cereal over the top, then press gently on the top of the cereal. Generously coat the cereal with canola cooking spray.

❖ Bake covered in oven for 30 minutes. Remove cover and bake an additional 10 to 15 minutes or until casserole is lightly browned on top and bubbling.

PER SERVING: 190 calories, 11.5 g protein, 14.5 g carbohydrate, 9 g fat (4.3 g saturated fat, 2.1 g monounsaturated fat, 1.8 g polyunsaturated fat), 29 mg cholesterol, 2.3 g fiber, 680 mg sodium. Calories from fat: 44 percent. Omega-3 fatty acids = 1.1 g Omega-6 fatty acids = .7 g Weight Watchers Winning Points = 4

Double-Decker Taco

MAKES 8 DOUBLE-DECKER TACOS

ॐ

One homemade double-decker taco contains half the fat and three times the fiber of two small crispy tacos from Taco Bell. Taco Bell featured these double-decker tacos on their menu, but for a limited time only. Now you can have them at home whenever the double-decker mood hits you—and they contain flaxseed.

Spicy beef filling:

1 pound super-lean ground beef (ground sirloin is fine)

¼ cup all-purpose flour

1 tablespoon chili powder

1 teaspoon salt

⅓ cup finely minced yellow or white onion

¼ teaspoon garlic powder

½ cup water

Canola cooking spray

¼ cup ground flaxseed

1 16-ounce can fat-free refried beans (Taco Bell brand is available in most supermarkets)

8 (soft taco size) flour tortillas

1 cup shredded reduced-fat cheddar cheese, for divided use

8 crispy taco shells (can be bought already made in boxes)

2 cups finely shredded iceberg lettuce

Taco sauce (Ortega or Taco Bell brand are available in bottles) optional

❖ In a large mixing bowl, add the ground beef, flour, chili powder, salt, onion, garlic powder, and water, and beat on lowest speed until well blended.

❖ Start heating a large nonstick frying pan or skillet over medium-high heat. Coat pan with canola cooking spray and add beef mixture. Cook mixture until brown, breaking up the meat into small pieces with a spatula while it cooks, about 6 minutes. The filling should end up being somewhat pasty without large chunks of beef. Stir in flaxseed.

❖ While beef is cooking, heat the refried beans in a small saucepan over medium-low heat, then stir in flaxseed.

❖ When beans and beef filling are ready, spread ⅛ cup of hot refried beans over the top of a flour tortilla and sprinkle with a tablespoon of the grated cheese. Wrap the prepared flour tortilla around a crispy corn taco shell and spoon ⅛ cup of the beef mixture inside the corn tortilla. Sprinkle with a tablespoon or two of grated cheese and ¼ cup of the shredded lettuce. Drizzle with taco sauce if desired. Repeat to assemble the remaining double-decker tacos.

PER DOUBLE-DECKER TACO: 370 calories, 23 g protein, 40 g carbohydrate, 13 g fat (5 g saturated fat, 3.7 g monounsaturated fat, 1.5 g polyunsaturated fat), 30 mg cholesterol, 6 g fiber, 810 mg sodium. Calories from fat: 32 percent. Omega-3 fatty acids = .8 g Omega-6 fatty acids = .5 g. Weight Watchers Winning Points = 8

Tamales Mini Pies

૨ว

I love tamales and sometimes I go all out, soaking cornhusks, filling, and fold-ing all of them—but steaming them for an hour in a big stock pot usually does me in. This year, a friend of mine told me that when she and her mother get tired of making tamales—when they get toward the bottom of the masa bowl— they start making tamale pies instead. So I thought, why not make tamale pies from the start? This way I get my tamale fix without too much trouble and I end up with a freezer full of potential quick lunch and dinner entrées too.

Filling:

4 roasted chicken breasts (remove skin) or 1 whole roasted or rotis-serie chicken (the kind you can buy at supermarkets)

1½ teaspoon canola oil

1 onion, chopped

1 teaspoon minced garlic (or 2 cloves, minced)

1 28-ounce can enchilada sauce (mild)

1 16-ounce can vegetarian or fat-free refried beans

½ cup ground flaxseed

Masa:

½ cup canola margarine (canola oil first ingredient)

½ cup fat-free or light sour cream

1 teaspoon chicken broth powder (optional)

1½ teaspoons salt (optional)

5½ cups chicken broth

6 cups masa harina de maiz (corn masa mix)

About 1 cup grated reduced-fat Jack or cheddar (optional)

❖ Preheat oven to 375°F. Cut chicken breasts into bite-sized pieces or shred pieces of all possible chicken meat from the chicken carcass (should be around 3 cups); set aside.

❖ Heat canola oil in medium nonstick frying pan. Add chopped onion and cook over medium heat, stirring frequently, until starting to brown. Stir in garlic and chicken pieces and let cook another minute. Reduce heat to medium-low and stir in enchilada sauce and beans and cook, stirring frequently until beans have blended in well. Remove from heat and stir in flaxseed.

❖ In a large mixing bowl, beat canola margarine, sour cream, salt, and chicken broth powder until fluffy. Add masa harina alternately with chicken broth to the margarine mixture in mixing bowl, mixing well after each addition. It will have the consistency of thick cake batter.

❖ Spread ¼ cup of masa mixture into bottom of each foil tart pan (or similar). Pour a heaping ¼ cup of chicken filling over the masa. Dot the top of the filling (or carefully spread) another ¼ cup of masa over the chicken and sauce.

❖ Bake for about 25 minutes until masa on top is lightly browned. Enjoy the tamale pies now, or freeze the tart pans in sealed plastic bags. To warm up, just invert tart pan on microwave-safe plate (lift and remove foil tart pan). Microwave on HIGH for 3 minutes or until warmed in center. Sprinkle grated cheese (cheddar or Jack) over the top and warm another minute in microwave, if desired.

PER MINI PIE: 312 calories, 14 g protein, 42 g carbohydrate, 10 g fat (3 g saturated fat, 3.7 g monounsaturated fat, 3.6 g polyunsaturated fat), 17 mg cholesterol, 7 g fiber, 572 mg sodium. Calories from fat: 29 percent. Omega-3 fatty acids = .7 g Omega-6 fatty acids = .4 g Weight Watchers Winning Points = 6

Pork Chimichangas

MAKES 9 CHIMICHANGAS

ʒ

The key to these lower-fat chimichangas is brushing the tortillas lightly with canola oil and then oven baking them to brown and crisp the outside instead of deep-frying them. You can freeze these in Ziploc freezer bags and just reheat in a toaster oven for a quick dinner or lunch.

2 tablespoons canola oil (more if needed), for divided use

1½ pounds pork tenderloin (about 2 small tenderloins), cut into 1-inch chunks (feel free to use the cracked pepper pork tenderloins that come vacuum packed and ready to roast in most supermarkets)

3 cups hot beef broth

2 tablespoons rice vinegar or distilled white vinegar

⅓ cup chopped green onion

⅓ cup finely chopped moderate chili peppers (such as Pasilla)

3 garlic cloves, minced (about ½ tablespoon)

1 teaspoon dried oregano, crumbled

½ teaspoon ground cumin

½ cup ground flaxseed

9–10 flour homestyle tortillas (baby burrito size works great)

1¼ cups vegetarian or nonfat canned refried beans (or similar)

Serve chimichangas with lime cilantro sauce and/or salsa (of your choice)

❖ In large, nonstick saucepan or skillet, add canola oil and spread with spatula. Heat over medium-high heat. Add pork tenderloin chunks and let brown on all sides (8 to 10 minutes).

❖ Meanwhile, start heating beef broth in a medium saucepan over medium heat. When pork tenderloins are nicely browned, add hot broth to the large saucepan with the pork, scraping the bottom of pan to loosen browned bits. Bring to a boil, then reduce heat to low. Cover and simmer until meat is tender, about 30 to 45 minutes.

❖ Preheat oven to 450° F. Uncover the pan, raise heat to high, and boil until over half of broth has evaporated, 8 to 10 minutes. Add in the vinegar, green onion, chili peppers, garlic, oregano, and cumin. Stir well and continue cooking until almost all of the broth has evaporated, about 5 minutes more). Stir in ground flaxseed. Let the pork cool completely, shredding the pork using a spatula or large spoon.

❖ Preheat oven to 450°F. Add a tablespoon of canola oil to a small dish.

❖ Heat each tortilla, one at a time, in a large, nonstick frying pan or skillet, following this method:

Heat one side of the tortilla until soft, then flip over to heat the other side while brushing the top lightly with canola oil using a pastry brush. Quickly flip oiled side of tortilla into a 9 × 13-inch baking dish. Spread ⅛ cup of refried beans in the middle of tortilla (spread it out to make a rectangle about 3 × 4 inches). Add ¼ cup of pork mixture over the top of beans. Fold in sides, then roll into a small compact burrito. Place seam-side down in the 9 × 13-inch baking dish.

❖ Repeat with remaining tortillas. Bake in center of oven for about 20 minutes or until both sides of chimichangas are nicely browned and crisp. Serve with lime-cilantro sauce (recipe below) and/or salsa if desired.

Lime-Cilantro Sauce:

1 cup nonfat or light sour cream

½ cup diced, peeled, and seeded cucumber

½ cup chopped fresh cilantro

1 tablespoon fresh lime juice

❖ Blend all ingredients in a food processor, pulsing, until cucumber is finely chopped and a nice sauce has formed. Season with salt and pepper if desired. Transfer to a serving bowl. You can prepare this an hour ahead of time—just keep it covered in the refrigerator until needed.

PER CHIMICHANGA: 360 calories, 25 g protein, 38 g carbohydrate, 12 g fat (2 g saturated fat, 5.3 g monounsaturated fat, 3.4 g polyunsaturated fat), 50 mg cholesterol, 4 g fiber, 828 mg sodium. Calories from fat: 31 percent. Omega-3 fatty acids = 1.6 g Omega-6 fatty acids = 1.7 g. Weight Watchers Winning Points = 7

Cajun Mini Meatloaves

MAKES 6 SERVINGS (2 CUPCAKE-SIZED MEATLOAVES EACH)

You'll never know there's flaxseed in these wonderfully moist meatloaves. This is my favorite way to give my husband his dose of flaxseed, because he doesn't even know he's getting it.

2 teaspoons canola oil

¼ cup nonalcoholic beer (regular beer or beef broth can be used)

⅔ cup finely chopped onions

½ cup finely chopped celery

½ cup finely chopped green or red bell peppers

¼ cup finely chopped green onions

2 teaspoons minced or chopped garlic (about 4 cloves)

2 teaspoons Tabasco sauce

2 teaspoons Creole or Cajun seasoning (add more if desired)

½ cup low-fat milk

½ cup ketchup

Canola cooking spray

1 pound ground sirloin or extra-lean ground beef

½ cup egg substitute

6 tablespoons ground flaxseed

½ cup very fine dry bread crumbs

2 ounces reduced-fat sharp cheddar, grated (about ½ cup) (optional)

❖ Add canola oil to large, nonstick saucepan or frying pan. Add beer, onions, celery, pepper, green onions, garlic, Tabasco, and Creole or Cajun seasoning blend to heated pan and sauté until the mixture starts sticking to the bottom of the pan (about 3 minutes), stirring frequently.

❖ Stir in milk and ketchup and continue cooking for about a minute, stirring occasionally. Remove from heat and let cool.

❖ Preheat oven to 350° F. Coat 12 muffin cups with canola cooking spray.

❖ Blend the ground beef, egg substitute, flaxseed, breadcrumbs, and ketchup and onion mixture, and ½ cup grated cheese (if desired) together using a spoon, your hands, or an electric mixer (use lowest speed).

❖ Fill prepared muffin cups with beef mixture and bake for about 15 to 20 minutes or until lightly browned and cooked throughout.

PER SERVING: 244 calories, 23 g protein, 17 g carbohydrate, 10 g fat (3 g saturated fat, 3 g monounsaturated fat, 2.7 g polyunsaturated fat), 48 mg cholesterol, 4 g fiber, 468 mg sodium. Calories from fat: 35 percent. Omega-3 fatty acids = 1.6 g Omega-6 fatty acids = .8 g. Weight Watchers Winning Points = 5

Light Sloppy Joes

MAKES 4 SLOPPY JOES

۽

Now you can enjoy delicious Sloppy Joe with less fat and lots of flax!

1 pound ground sirloin (or extra lean ground beef)

½ cup chopped onion

½ cup chopped green bell pepper

½ teaspoon garlic powder

1 tablespoon prepared mustard

¾ cup plus 2 tablespoons ketchup

½ cup water

2 tablespoons brown sugar, packed

½ teaspoon salt (optional)

½ teaspoon pepper (add more to taste)

¼ cup ground flaxseed

4 hamburger buns (or similar)

grated reduced-fat Monterey Jack or cheddar cheese (optional)

❖ Brown ground sirloin, onion, and green pepper over medium heat in large, nonstick frying pan or skillet.

❖ Stir in the garlic powder, mustard, ketchup, water, brown sugar; mix thoroughly. Reduce heat, cover, and let simmer for 20 minutes, stirring every 5 minutes or so. Add salt (optional), pepper, flaxseed, and stir. Serve ¼ of mixture over a hamburger bun or similar (open faced or fitted together). Sprinkle each with a tablespoon or two of cheese if desired.

PER SLOPPY JOE: 390 calories, 28.5 g protein, 50.5 g carbohydrate, 10 g fat (3 g saturated fat, 3 g monounsaturated fat, 3.4 g polyunsaturated fat), 60 mg cholesterol, 5.3 g fiber, 990 mg sodium. Calories from fat: 23 percent. Omega-3 fatty acids = 1.6 g Omega-6 fatty acids = 1.3 g. Weight Watchers Winning Points = 8

Microwave Mini Lasagna

ॐ

The added chicken broth in the spaghetti sauce helps "boil" the noodles while the lasagna cooks. After trying this recipe, you may never boil lasagna noodles again! If you want to add your vegetable serving in, just stir two cups of lightly cooked carrot coins or chopped broccoli florets into the cheese mixture. It will add a couple grams of fiber to each serving and a big boost of antioxidants. Since this recipe is designed to make one loaf pan of lasagna, you can double it easily to make two loaf pans (six servings).

1½ cups bottled spaghetti sauce of your choice

½ cup vegetable or chicken broth

3 tablespoons ground flaxseed

½ cup part-skim or low-fat ricotta cheese

⅓ cup plus ⅛ cup grated part-skim mozzarella cheese, packed

3 tablespoons grated Parmesan cheese, divided

2 green onions, chopped

1 tablespoon chopped fresh parsley or 1 teaspoon dried parsley

1 tablespoon chopped fresh basil leaves or 1 teaspoon dried basil (optional)

1½ tablespoons egg substitute

⅛ teaspoon salt (optional)

Dash of pepper

Canola cooking spray

6 wide lasagna noodles (uncooked), about 7 ounces

❖ Stir spaghetti sauce, broth, and ground flaxseed in a 4-cup measure and set aside.

❖ In medium bowl, combine ricotta, ⅓ cup mozzarella, 2 tablespoons Parmesan, green onion, parsley, basil, egg substitute, salt, and pepper.

❖ Spray 9 × 5-inch glass loaf pan with canola or olive oil cooking spray. Layer ½ cup spaghetti sauce mixture in loaf pan, then 2 strips of uncooked noodles (breaking them to fit). Dot the noodles with ⅓ of the cheese mixture. Cover the cheese with ½-cup spaghetti sauce and 2 more strips of noodles. Dot the noodles with another third of the cheese mixture. Top the cheese with ½ cup spaghetti sauce and the 2 last noodles. Spread the remaining ½ cup of sauce over the top and sprinkle the remaining Parmesan and mozzarella over the top.

❖ Spray one side of microwave-safe plastic wrap with cooking spray (so the cheese doesn't stick to the wrap) and use it to cover the lasagna tightly.

Microwave on HIGH for 25 minutes. Rotate dish a quarter turn every 10 minutes or so. Let stand 10 minutes before cutting.

PER SERVING: 435 calories, 24 g protein, 57.5 g carbohydrate, 12 g fat (5.4 g saturated fat, 3.1 g monounsaturated fat, 2.6 g polyunsaturated fat), 26 mg cholesterol, 4.5 g fiber, 468 mg sodium. Calories from fat: 25 percent. Omega-3 fatty acids = 1.6 g Omega-6 fatty acids = 1 g. Weight Watchers Winning Points = 9

Oriental Chicken Wraps

ॐ

The contrast between cold and crispy lettuce wrapped around warm and savory chicken and vegetables is simply irresistible.

2 teaspoons light soy sauce

4 teaspoons dry sherry (chicken broth can be substituted)

1 teaspoon sesame oil

1 teaspoon cornstarch

2 large (or 3 small) boneless and skinless chicken breasts

2 teaspoons canola oil

4 large garlic cloves, chopped (about 2 teaspoons)

1 tablespoon finely chopped fresh ginger

3 whole green onions, chopped

½ cup finely chopped carrot (about 1 carrot)

½ cup finely chopped celery (about 1 stalk)

2 tablespoons bottled hoisin sauce

2 tablespoons bottled plum sauce (you'll find both sauces in the Asian food section of your supermarket)

¼ cup ground flaxseed

8 large leaves iceberg lettuce, rinsed and dried well

½ cup crunchy canned chow mein noodles (optional)

❖ Mix soy sauce, sherry (or broth), sesame oil, and cornstarch in 2-cup measure.

❖ Place chicken breasts in food processor. Drizzle the marinade over the top and process mixture until chicken looks like ground pork. Spoon mixture back into the 2-cup measure, cover, and refrigerate for at least 30 minutes.

❖ Heat nonstick skillet or large frying pan on medium heat. Add canola oil, garlic, and ginger and cook about 10 seconds. Add chicken mixture, breaking lumps into small pieces with pancake turner until chicken is cooked through, about 6 minutes.

❖ Add chopped vegetables; toss for 1 minute or until tender-crisp. Stir in hoisin sauce, plum sauce, and flaxseed; toss to mix.

❖ Spoon ⅛ of chicken mixture into center of each lettuce leaf and sprinkle with a tablespoon of chow mein noodles. Eat this with your hands!

PER SERVING: 201 calories, 16 g protein, 15 g carbohydrates, 8 g fat (1 g saturated fat, 2.6 g monounsaturated fat, 3.1 g polyunsaturated fat), 36 mg cholesterol, 4 g fiber, 388 mg sodium. Calories from fat: 36 percent. Omega-3 fatty acids = 1.8 g Omega-6 fatty acids = 1.3 g Weight Watchers Winning Points = 4

Chicken and Rice Salad

MAKES 4 LARGE SALAD SERVINGS

၁၅

You can save time by buying a roasted chicken at the supermarket or nearby rotisserie. Dicing up the two skinless breast portions will give you exactly the amount of chicken you need for this recipe.

4 teaspoons lemon juice

¾ cup fat-free or light sour cream

1 tablespoon real mayonnaise

¼ teaspoon poultry seasoning

Couple of dashes ground black pepper

1 tablespoon green olive juice (from bottle of sliced green olives)

3 cups cooked long-grain brown* or white rice, cooled

2 cups diced cooked/roasted chicken breast, skinless

1 cup diced celery

½ cup sliced green olives

¼ cup sliced almonds plus 2 tablespoons (if desired), toasted (toast in oven until lightly browned)

¼ cup sliced green onions (white and part of green)

¼ cup ground flaxseed

Salt to taste

❖ Add lemon juice, sour cream, mayonnaise, poultry seasoning, pepper, and green olive juice to large mixing bowl. Beat on low until creamy and well blended.

❖ Add remaining ingredients to mixing bowl and toss to mix all of the ingredients together with the dressing. Add salt and more pepper to taste and sprinkle 2 tablespoons of extra sliced almonds (toasted) over the top before serving if desired.

*To cook brown rice, bring 2 cups of water and ½ teaspoon salt to boil in small saucepan. Add 1 cup of brown rice, cover, and return to boil. Reduce heat to simmer and let cook for about 1 hour (do not lift lid during this time). Remove from heat and use a fork to fluff.

PER SALAD SERVING: 395 calories, 23 g protein, 47 g carbohydrate, 13 g fat (2.2 g saturated fat, 5 g monounsaturated fat, 5 g polyunsaturated fat), 42 mg cholesterol, 6.3 g fiber, 330 mg sodium. Calories from fat: 30 percent. Omega-3 fatty acids = 1.5 g Omega-6 fatty acids = 1.9 g. Weight Watchers Winning Points = 8

Three-Step Taco Salad

MAKES 4 TO 6 SERVINGS

This taco salad is quick to make and a treat to eat on hot summer days. You decide how spicy you want the dressing by choosing mild, medium, or hot salsa. I've cut down on the ground beef a bit in this recipe and added some beans to give it a fiber and nutrition boost.

1 pound ground sirloin (or extra-lean ground beef)

1 packet (1.25 oz) taco seasoning

¼ cup ground flaxseed

⅔ cup fat-free or light sour cream

⅔ cup bottled salsa (choose mild, medium, or hot, depending on preference)

8 cups shredded iceberg lettuce (other lettuce types can be used)

2 cups chopped tomatoes, drained

1 15-ounce can low-sodium kidney or black beans, rinsed and drained

½ cup grated reduced-fat sharp cheddar cheese, packed

4 ounces (about 4 cups) bite-size tortilla chips ("baked" or reduced-fat tortilla chips can also be used)

1 avocado, pitted, peeled, and cut into thin strips for garnish (optional)

sliced black olives for garnish (optional)

Grated, reduced-fat sharp cheddar cheese for garnish (optional)

❖ Add taco seasoning packet to browned ground beef in nonstick frying pan. Pour in ¾ cup water and bring to boil, reduce heat and simmer 5 minutes, stirring occasionally. Stir in flaxseed and set aside to cool.

❖ Add sour cream and salsa to small or medium mixing bowl and beat until blended well; set aside.

❖ Add lettuce, tomatoes, beans, cheese, tortilla chips, and cooled sirloin mixture to large serving bowl. Drizzle desired amount of dressing over the top and toss to blend well. Garnish with extra grated cheese, black olives, and avocado strips (if desired) and serve.

PER SERVING (IF 6 SERVINGS): 380 calories, 28 g protein, 40 g carbohydrate, 12.5 g fat (3.8 g saturated fat, 1.9 g monounsaturated fat, 2.2 g polyunsaturated fat), 49 mg cholesterol, 11 g fiber, 800 mg sodium. Calories from fat: 28 percent. Omega-3 fatty acids = 1.14 g Omega-6 fatty acids = .43 g. Weight Watchers Winning Points = 7

Chicken Flautas

MAKES 24 FLAUTAS

༄

I bake these chicken flautas instead of deep-frying them, so now you can enjoy this delicious Mexican dish without all the extra fat.

4 cups skinless, boneless, roasted
  chicken breast, shredded
4 green onions, white and part of
  green, chopped
1 8-ounce jar green taco sauce (mild)
¼ teaspoon ground cumin (optional)
8 ounces shredded reduced-fat
  Monterey Jack cheese (or mixture
  of reduced-fat Colby and Jack)
24 corn tortillas
Canola cooking spray
up to 4 tablespoons ground flaxseed
  (about ½ teaspoon per flauta)

SERVING SUGGESTIONS: Serve with guacamole, jalapeño jelly, or fat-free or light sour cream for dipping.

PER SERVING (3 FLAUTAS PER SERVING): 397 calories, 31 g protein, 42 g carbohydrate, 12.5 g fat (5 g saturated fat, 1.8 g monounsaturated fat, 3.1 g polyunsaturated fat), 68 mg cholesterol, 7 g fiber, 591 mg sodium. Calories from fat: 28 percent. Omega-3 fatty acids = 1.5 g Omega-6 fatty acids = 1.5 g. Weight Watchers Winning Points: 8

❖ Preheat oven to 350° F. In a medium bowl, combine shredded chicken, green onions, green taco sauce, cumin, and cheese and mix together well.

❖ Start heating small, nonstick skillet over medium heat.

❖ Add one tortilla and let heat about a minute. Spray the top lightly with canola cooking spray and flip over briefly. Place softened tortilla in a 9 × 13-inch baking pan (you'll need two pans altogether), canola-oil-spray-side down. While you are filling this tortilla you can add another tortilla to the pan to soften.

❖ Place ⅛ cup of chicken mixture down the tortilla about ⅓ of the way from one end. Sprinkle ½ teaspoon of flaxseed down the center of the tortillas. Wrap up tightly and place seam-side down in the pan.

❖ Repeat steps 3 and 4 until all the tortillas are filled or the chicken mixture is gone (whichever comes first).

❖ Bake for about 20 to 25 minutes or until tortillas are a little crispy and golden brown.

Cheese Enchiladas with Green Chiles

MAKES 8 ENCHILADAS (ABOUT 4 SERVINGS)

✌

If you aren't crazy about chili peppers, just make some of the enchiladas without them. Dress each enchilada with a drizzle of mild green taco sauce (available at the supermarket), a dollop of sour cream, and a black olive just before serving. Garnish each plate with a slice or two of avocado.

1 16-ounce bottle mild enchilada sauce

4 green onions, chopped (white and
    part of green)

2 cups shredded reduced-fat Colby or
    Monterey Jack cheese (or similar)

8 6½-inch corn tortillas

1 cup of canned fat-free refried beans
    (or vegetarian)

¼ cup ground flaxseed (golden flax
    works best in this recipe)

1 7-ounce can Ortega mild whole
    green chili

½ cup tacqueria-style mild green taco
    sauce

½ cup nonfat or light sour cream

8 black olives, pitted (optional)

1 avocado, sliced (optional)

PER SERVING (2 ENCHILADAS PER SERVING): 450 calories, 25 g protein, 59 g carbohydrate, 12.5 g fat (6.3 g saturated fat, 3.5 g monounsaturated fat, 2.8 g poly-unsaturated fat), 32 mg cholesterol, 11 g fiber, 992 mg sodium. Calories from fat: 25 percent. Omega-3 fatty acids = 1.7 g Omega-6 fatty acids = 2 g. Weight Watchers Winning Points = 9

❖ Preheat oven to 400° F. Add enchilada sauce to bottom of 9 × 13-inch pan.

❖ Add green onions and shredded cheese to medium-size bowl and toss to blend well.

❖ Wrap corn tortillas in a damp kitchen towel and heat in microwave until tortillas are soft, about 2 minutes. Meanwhile, heat beans in small saucepan over medium-low heat and stir in flaxseed.

❖ Spread ⅛ cup of bean/flaxseed mixture down the center of each tortilla and sprinkle about ⅓ cup of cheese mixture over top. Lay a strip of chiles on top of the cheese and roll up. Lay enchilada down in pan, seam-side up, then turn enchilada over so it is seam side down and the tortilla is coated with sauce. Repeat with remaining tortillas, cheese, and chiles.

❖ Bake, covered, for 12 minutes. Remove cover; bake for extra 5 minutes or until heated through and cheese is melted.

❖ Dress each enchilada with a drizzle of mild green taco sauce (available in bottles), a dollop of sour cream, and a black olive. Garnish each plate with a slice or two of avocado.

Ranger Rick Ranch Beans

MAKES 6 TO 8 ENTRÉE SERVINGS

༨

This is a satisfying and savory dish that can be served on the side at a barbeque or potluck or as the main dish with rolls, cornbread, or fruit salad. Since the sauce is so dark, you don't even notice the flaxseed is in there.

1 28-ounce can baked beans (I use Maple Cured Bacon Bush's baked beans)

1 medium onion, diced

1 medium bell pepper, diced

1 14-ounce package Louis Rich Turkey Polska Kielbasa sausage links (or similar lower-fat sausage), cut into small, bite-sized chunks

½ cup ketchup

1 14½-ounce can diced tomatoes, well drained (you can leave this out if desired)

1–2 tablespoons chili powder (use 1 tablespoon for a kid-friendly version)

3 tablespoons Worcestershire sauce

3 tablespoons apple cider vinegar (or white vinegar)

½ cup packed brown sugar

1 tablespoon minced or chopped garlic (1 teaspoon garlic powder can be substituted)

Salt to taste

1 or 2 dashes cayenne pepper (add more to taste)

1 tablespoon red pepper flakes (optional—if you want to turn up the "heat")

6 tablespoons ground flaxseed

❖ Add baked beans, diced onion, bell pepper, sausage, ketchup, and diced stewed tomatoes to slow cooker.

❖ Sprinkle chili powder, Worcestershire sauce, vinegar, brown sugar, garlic, salt if desired, and cayenne pepper over the top of bean mixture and stir well.

❖ Turn slow cooker on HIGH and heat 2 to 4 hours or turn slow cooker on LOW and heat 8 to 10 hours. Spoon into serving bowls and stir in ½ tablespoon to 1 tablespoon flaxseed per serving.

NOTE: If you want to use a Dutch oven, preheat oven to 350°F, add all the ingredients to Dutch oven, stir, and bake for 1 hour.

PER SERVING: 308 calories, 15 g protein, 49 g carbohydrate, 8 g fat (1.4 g saturated fat, 2 g monounsaturated fat, 2.6 g poly-unsaturated fat), 32 mg cholesterol, 8 g fiber, 762 mg sodium. Calories from fat: 23 percent. Omega-3 fatty acids = 1.2 g Omega-6 fatty acids = 1.4 g. Weight Watchers Winning Points = 6

Stuffed Red Bell Peppers

These tasty peppers can be made to order. If you want to keep them vegetarian, leave out the light sausage. If the red peppers are too expensive, use green bell peppers. If you want to pump up the fiber and nutrients, use brown rice instead of white.

3 large red bell peppers (green, yellow, or orange can be substituted)

1 tablespoon olive oil

1 cup chopped onions

1 portobello mushroom, chopped (about 1 cup) crimini or regular mushrooms can be substituted

3 tablespoons chopped fresh parsley

2 teaspoons minced or chopped garlic

5 ounces (about 1 cup) Light Jimmy Dean sausage, chopped (super-lean ground beef or Lite turkey Polska Kielbasa, chopped, can be substituted)

1½ cups cooked white or brown rice

½ teaspoon paprika (add more to taste if desired)

½ teaspoon salt

½ teaspoon ground black pepper

⅛ teaspoon ground allspice

1 cup bottled marinara sauce (tomato sauce can be substituted)

3 tablespoons ground flaxseed

⅓ cup grated reduced-fat sharp cheddar cheese (optional)

❖ Cut the tops off the peppers (reserve tops) and scoop the seeds and inside flesh from them. Discard the stems but chop the pepper tops and set aside. Add peppers to large microwave-safe dish with about a cup of water in the bottom, cover, and microwave on HIGH until just tender, about 8 minutes. Remove peppers from the water and set aside to cool.

❖ Meanwhile, heat oil in small or medium non-stick frying pan over medium-high heat. Add onions, mushrooms, parsley, garlic, and reserved chopped pepper pieces. Sauté mixture, stirring often, until onions are softened, about 4 to 6 minutes. Spoon into a large bowl.

❖ Add light sausage, lean beef, or turkey polska kielbasa to the same frying pan and cook over medium heat, crumbling with spatula as it cooks, until nicely brown and cooked through, about 5 minutes. Add to onion mixture in bowl, along with the cooked rice, paprika, salt, pepper, allspice, ½ cup of the marinara sauce, and the flaxseed. Stir to blend ingredients well.

❖ Fill the peppers with the rice mixture and stand the filled peppers in a loaf pan or similar deep dish and microwave on HIGH about 8 minutes more. Pour remaining marinara evenly over the tops of the peppers and sprinkle with cheese, if desired. Microwave, uncovered, 2 to 3 minutes more.

NOTE: These can be made one day ahead. Just cover, chill, and rewarm in microwave or oven.

PER PEPPER: 360 calories, 14 g protein, 51 g carbohydrate, 12 g fat (2.1 g saturated fat, 5.7 g monounsaturated fat, 4.2 g polyunsaturated fat), 24 mg cholesterol, 10 g fiber, 946 mg sodium. Calories from fat: 30 percent. Omega-3 fatty acids = 1.6 g Omega-6 fatty acids = 1.8 g. Weight Watchers Winning Points = 7

Eggplant Parmesan with Roasted Red Peppers and Caramelized Onions

MAKES 3 SERVINGS (TO MAKE 6 SERVINGS,
JUST DOUBLE THE RECIPE AND USE AN 8 x 8-INCH BAKING DISH)

Eggplant Parmesan is one of my favorite non-meat dishes. It's savory, it's cheesy, and you probably won't even miss the meat. I add a layer of roasted red peppers and caramelized onion slices for a little extra flavor and nutrients. You can double the recipe and make two loaf pans—freeze one for one of those hectic weeknights.

Canola or olive oil cooking spray

1 medium eggplant (about 1 pound)

½ cup egg substitute (or 2 eggs, beaten)

⅔ cup unseasoned breadcrumbs (French or similar)

½ teaspoon seasoning salt

¾ teaspoon garlic powder with parsley

¼ teaspoon black pepper

2 teaspoons olive oil (flavored olive oils can be used, if desired)

½ large onion, sliced

1½ cups bottled marinara sauce

3 tablespoons ground flaxseed

½ cup roasted red pepper strips (half of a 7¼-ounce jar)

½ cup shredded part-skim mozzarella cheese, packed

6 tablespoons shredded Parmesan cheese

Fresh parsley for garnish, if desired.

❖ Preheat oven to 375° F. Coat a 9-inch loaf pan with canola or olive oil cooking spray.

❖ Cut eggplant crosswise into slices about ¼-inch thick. Add egg substitute to a shallow bowl. Add breadcrumbs, seasoning salt, garlic powder, and black pepper to a second shallow bowl and blend well.

❖ Dip each eggplant slice in egg substitute (covering both sides well), then in the breadcrumb mixture (coating both sides well) and set on a plate or wax paper.

❖ Begin heating a large, nonstick frying pan over medium heat. Coat the bottom with a teaspoon of the olive oil and distribute half of the slices evenly in pan. Coat the tops of the eggplant slices with canola or olive oil cooking spray. Once the bottom is lightly browned, flip slices over and brown other side.

❖ Remove slices from pan and repeat Step 4 with remaining olive oil and eggplant slices.

❖ Start heating a small, nonstick frying pan over medium heat. Coat bottom with canola or olive oil cooking spray and add onion slices. Coat tops of onion slices with cooking spray. When underside is brown, flip over and brown other side. Remove pan from heat.

❖ Add 3 eggplant slices to prepared loaf pan and cover with ½ cup of the marinara sauce. Sprinkle with 3 tablespoons of Parmesan and the flaxseed. Top with the roasted red pepper strips and caramelized onion slices. Top with 3 more eggplant slices, then cover the top with the remaining marinara sauce, the mozzarella cheese, and the remaining Parmesan.

❖ Bake, covered, for 25 minutes or until cheese and sauce is bubbling. Let rest 10 minutes before serving. Garnish with parsley, if desired.

NOTE: If you want to use seasoned breadcrumbs, just omit the seasoning salt, garlic powder, and black pepper.

PER SERVING: 337 calories, 18 g protein, 34 g carbohydrate, 14 g fat (5 g saturated fat, 5.2 g monounsaturated fat, 3.8 g polyunsaturated fat), 17 mg cholesterol, 10 g fiber, 914 mg sodium. Calories from fat: 37 percent. Omega-3 fatty acids = 1.6 g Omega-6 fatty acids = .8 g. Weight Watchers Winning Points = 7

9

Decadent Desserts

Some might say it is nutritional sacrilege to add flaxseed to a dessert recipe; that flaxseed, if it had any say, would never be caught dead on the same page as decadent, nutritionally void items such as sugar or chocolate. All those in favor of this traditional way of thinking, turn back to chapters 1 through 8 while you still have a chance. And for all those opposed, who like to take risks in the kitchen, who like to have their cake and flaxseed, too—read on.

You just won't believe you are getting your flaxseed allotment when you eat these tasty treats. Mind you, some of these recipes have more going for them nutritionally than others—some contain other whole grains or fruit servings while others are just packed with sugar and chocolate. But I personally don't let a day go by without a little bite of chocolate. From Peach Raspberry Fruit Crisp and Kahlua Chocolate Fudge Cake to Chewy Oatmeal Raisin Bites and Key Lime Parfait, trust me, you will be looking forward to getting your daily dose of flaxseed.

Oatmeal-Raisin Bites

MAKES ABOUT 76 BITES (MINI COOKIES)

જી

I absolutely love these cookies because they have the taste and texture of regular, high-fat oatmeal cookies.

Canola cooking spray

5 tablespoons butter or canola margarine, softened

3 tablespoons light or fat-free cream cheese

½ cup packed brown sugar

¼ cup white sugar

1 large egg (or ¼ cup egg substitute)

½ cup ground flaxseed

½ cup unbleached flour

½ teaspoon baking soda

½ teaspoon salt

2 teaspoons vanilla extract

1 cup baking raisins (regular raisins will work, too)

¾ cup quick-cooking oats

❖ Preheat oven to 375° F. Coat double thickness cookie sheets with canola cooking spray.

❖ In mixing bowl, cream together butter, cream cheese, and sugars. Add egg and beat well.

❖ Add flaxseed, flour, baking soda, salt, and vanilla to butter mixture and beat until well blended. Stir in raisins and oats. Blend thoroughly.

❖ Drop rounded teaspoons of dough onto cookie sheet (about 20 bites per cookie sheet). Bake in center of oven for about 6 minutes or until cookies are still soft but lightly browned. Remove cookies and let cool on wire rack.

PER 4 BITES (4 MINI COOKIES): 130 calories, 2.5 g protein, 21 g carbohydrate, 4.7 g fat (2 g saturated fat, 1.3 g monounsaturated fat, 1 g polyunsaturated fat), 19 mg cholesterol, 2 g fiber, 84 mg sodium. Calories from fat: 32 percent. Omega-3 fatty acids = .7 g Omega-6 fatty acids = .3 g. Weight Watchers Winning Points = 3

Double Chocolate Cake-Mix Cookies

MAKES 24 LARGE, BAKERY-SIZE COOKIES

These fudgy cookies are wonderfully moist and chewy—like little miniature chocolate cakes—and a cinch to make.

1 box Betty Crocker Super Moist Devil's Food cake mix

3 tablespoons butter or canola margarine, softened

⅓ cup fat-free sour cream (light sour cream can be substituted)

2 teaspoons vanilla extract

1 egg

¼ cup egg substitute (or 2 egg whites)

½ cup ground flaxseed

1 cup semisweet or white chocolate chips (optional)

❖ Preheat oven to 350°F. Beat 2 cups of the dry cake mix, the butter, sour cream, vanilla, egg, and egg substitute in large mixing bowl on medium speed until smooth (or mix well with spoon).

❖ Stir in remaining cake mix, the flaxseed, and chocolate chips. Drop by cookie scoop (or rounded tablespoons) about 2 inches apart onto cookie sheet coated with canola cooking spray or lined with parchment paper.

❖ Bake 10 to 12 minutes or until edges are set (centers will be soft). Cool 1 minute; remove from cookie sheet to wire rack.

PER COOKIE (WITH CHOCOLATE CHIPS): 132 calories, 2 g protein, 19 g carbohydrate, 5.5 g fat (3 g saturated fat, 1.7 g monounsaturated fat, .6 g polyunsaturated fat), 13 mg cholesterol, 1.2 g fiber, 150 mg sodium. Calories from fat: 38 percent. Omega-3 fatty acids = .4 g Omega-6 fatty acids = .2 g. Weight Watchers Winning Points = 3

Pumpkin Spice Flaxseed Cookies

MAKES 28 LARGE COOKIES

ॐ

I have to admit—these cookies taste so good and are so nutritious I some-times even eat them for breakfast.

Canola cooking spray

¼ cup granulated sugar

¼ cup dark brown sugar, packed

½ cup butter or canola margarine, softened

½ cup honey

1 cup canned pumpkin (unsweetened)

2 teaspoons vanilla extract

1 large egg

2 cups flour

1 teaspoon baking powder

1 teaspoon baking soda

1 teaspoon ground cinnamon

¼ teaspoon salt

¾ cup ground flaxseed

28 pecan halves (optional)

❖ Preheat oven to 350°F and coat cookie sheet with canola cooking spray.

❖ Add sugar, brown sugar, butter, and honey to mixing bowl and beat until light and fluffy.

❖ Add the pumpkin, vanilla, and egg to sugar mixture in mixing bowl and beat until blended.

❖ Add flour, baking powder, baking soda, cinnamon, and salt to 8-cup measure (or medium-sized bowl) and stir to blend. Add it all at once to the pumpkin mixture in mixing bowl, and beat on low until blended (scraping sides of bowl midway). Stir in the flaxseed by hand.

❖ Drop the dough by cookie scoop (or rounded tablespoon) onto prepared cookie sheet. Press pecan half in the center of each cookie (this will help flatten the cookie). If you aren't adding a pecan half, flatten each cookie a little with your fingers (it will be a bit sticky). Bake about 11 to 12 minutes. Remove cookies from cookie sheet.

PER COOKIE (WITH PECAN HALF): 122 calories, 2 g protein, 17 g carbohydrate, 5.3 g fat (2.3 g saturated fat, 1.8 g monounsaturated fat, 1.2 g polyunsaturated fat), 16 mg cholesterol, 1.6 g fiber, 58 mg sodium. Calories from fat: 38 percent. Omega-3 fatty acids = .7 g Omega-6 fatty acids = .5 g. Weight Watchers Winning Points = 2

PER COOKIE (WITHOUT PECAN HALF): 112 calories, 2 g protein, 16.5 g carbohydrate, 4.4 g fat (2.2 g saturated fat, 1.3 g monounsaturated fat, .9 g polyunsaturated fat), 16 mg cholesterol, 1.5 g fiber, 58 mg sodium. Calories from fat: 35 percent. Omega-3 fatty acids = .7 g Omega-6 fatty acids = .2 g. Weight Watchers Winning Points = 2

Honey Bun Cake

ॐ

This is a light version of a Betty Crocker Most Requested Recipe. If you can't find the flaxseed, that's because it's hidden in the cinnamon-sugar middle part.

3 tablespoons butter or canola margarine, softened

1 package Betty Crocker Super Moist Butter Recipe Yellow Cake Mix

1 cup pureed peaches* (about 2 peaches)

2 large eggs

½ cup egg substitute

1⅛ cup nonfat or light sour cream

½ cup packed brown sugar

⅓ cup chopped pecans

2 teaspoons ground cinnamon

½ cup ground flaxseed

Icing:

1 cup powdered sugar

1 tablespoon milk (any type), and more as needed

1 teaspoon vanilla extract

❖ Preheat oven to 350°F. Generously grease bottom only of 13 × 9-inch pan with butter or canola margarine. Remove ½ of the dry cake mix (about 2 cups); reserve for later.

❖ Beat remaining dry cake mix, butter, peach puree, eggs, egg substitute, and sour cream in large mixing bowl on medium speed for 2 minutes, scraping bowl occasionally.

❖ Spread half of the batter in the prepared pan.

❖ In 2-cup measure, stir together reserved dry cake mix, brown sugar, pecans, cinnamon, and flaxseed; sprinkle evenly over the batter in pan.

❖ Carefully spread remaining batter evenly over cinnamon-sugar mixture by dropping batter by dollops over the mixture, then spreading. Bake 30 to 33 minutes or until cake springs back when touched lightly in center.

*Puree peaches by taking peach slices and pulsing in food processor or mashing well with potato masher.

❖ For icing, stir powdered sugar, milk, and vanilla until thin enough to drizzle, stirring in additional milk, 1 teaspoon at a time, if necessary. Poke top of warm cake several times with fork, then spread icing over top. Cool completely, about 1 hour. Store covered.

PER SLICE: 373 calories, 6.5 g protein, 62 g carbohydrate, 11 g fat (3.5 g saturated fat, 2.9 g monounsaturated fat, 2.2 g polyunsaturated fat), 45 mg cholesterol, 2.2 g fiber, 372 mg sodium. Calories from fat: 26 percent. Omega-3 fatty acids = 1.1 g Omega-6 fatty acids = 1.1 g. Weight Watchers Winning Points = 8

Chewy Chocolate Chip Flax Cookies

MAKES 18 LARGE COOKIES

This wouldn't be a dessert chapter without a recipe for chocolate chip cookies. Hot from the oven, there's nothing better.

4 tablespoons butter, room temperature (canola margarine can also be used)

¼ cup reduced-calorie pancake syrup or maple syrup

½ cup packed brown sugar

¼ cup granulated sugar

1 teaspoon vanilla extract

2 tablespoons beaten egg (2 tablespoons of egg substitute can also be used)

1 cup flour

¼ teasoon baking soda

¼ teaspoon salt

¾ cup semisweet chocolate chips (a combination of semisweet and white chocolate chips can also be used)

⅓ cup ground flaxseed

❖ Preheat oven to 375°F. Line two baking sheets with parchment paper or coat with canola cooking spray and set aside.

❖ Combine butter, syrup, and both sugars in mixing bowl and beat until light and fluffy, about 1 minute, scraping bowl in between. Add vanilla and egg and continue beating until well combined.

❖ In a medium bowl, whisk together flour, baking soda, and salt. Slowly add to the butter mixture, mixing on low speed until just combined. Stir in chocolate chips and flaxseed.

❖ Fill a level cookie scoop (about 2 tablespoons of dough) and place each on the prepared baking sheets. Place scoops 3 inches apart because the dough will spread out.

❖ Bake until just brown around the edges, about 15 minutes. Remove from oven and let cool slightly before removing cookies to a wire rack. Store in airtight container at room temperature for up to one week.

PER COOKIE: 125 calories, 2 g protein, 19 g carbohydrate, 5 g fat (2.5 g saturated fat), 7 mg cholesterol, 2 g fiber, 90 mg sodium. Calories from fat: 34 percent. Omega-3 fatty acids = .5 g Omega-6 fatty acids = .2 g. Weight Watchers Points = 2

Best Blueberry Coffee Cake

MAKES 8 SERVINGS

ᒎ

This cake couldn't be any better—it's moist, full of flavor, and you can hide the flaxseed in the crumb topping.

Canola cooking spray

2 cups cake flour (regular can be substituted)

½ cup plus ⅛ cup granulated sugar

2½ teaspoons baking powder

¾ teaspoon salt

3 tablespoons canola oil

2 tablespoons honey (light corn syrup can be substituted)

¾ cup low-fat milk

1 large egg

2 cups fresh or frozen blueberries

Crumb topping:

½ cup granulated sugar

¼ cup ground flaxseed

2 tablespoons flour

¾ teaspoon ground cinnamon

2 tablespoons butter or canola margarine, softened

2 tablespoons fat-free or light sour cream

Glaze:

½ cup powdered sugar

¼ teaspoon vanilla extract

1½ to 2 teaspoons hot water

❖ Preheat oven to 375°F. Coat a 9 × 9 × 2 square or round cake pan with canola cooking spray.

❖ Add the first 8 ingredients to mixing bowl and beat for about 30 seconds until blended. Carefully stir in blueberries and spread in prepared pan.

❖ Add the crumb topping ingredients to a small food processor (or use pastry blender and a medium-sized bowl) and mix together briefly—just until blended and crumbly. Sprinkle topping evenly over cake batter.

❖ Bake 45 minutes in center of oven or until cake tests done.

❖ Meanwhile, add glaze ingredients to 2-cup measure and mix until smooth and of drizzling consistency. Drizzle finished cake with glaze and serve coffee cake warm or cool.

PER SERVING: 375 calories, 5 g protein, 67 g carbohydrate, 9 g fat (2.7 g saturated fat, 4.5 g monounsaturated fat, 2.9 g polyunsaturated fat), 36 mg cholesterol, 3 g fiber, 407 mg sodium. Calories from fat: 23 percent. Omega-3 fatty acids = 1.3 g Omega-6 fatty acids = 1.5 g. Weight Watchers Winning Points = 8

Rocky Road Brownies

MAKES 18 LARGE SERVINGS

೨෮

Get ready, because these will be a new family favorite, pleasing kids and die-hard chocolate addicts alike.

Canola cooking spray

1 box (18¼ ounces) German chocolate cake mix (I use Betty Crocker Super Moist)

3 tablespoons canola oil

¼ cup chocolate syrup

⅔ cup evaporated skimmed or low-fat milk (not sweetened condensed)

1/2 cup ground flaxseed

Frosting:

2 tablespoons butter, softened

3 tablespoons chocolate syrup

⅔ cup cocoa

1 teaspoon vanilla extract

2 cups powdered sugar

¼ cup evaporated skim or low-fat milk

2 cups miniature marshmallows

½ cup walnut pieces to sprinkle on top (optional)

PER SERVING: 270 calories, 4.5 g protein, 48 g carbohydrate, 7 g fat (2.5 g saturated fat, 3.0 g monounsaturated fat, 1.5 g poly-unsaturated fat), 11 mg cholesterol, 2.5 g fiber, 243 mg sodium. Calories from fat: 26 percent. Omega-3 fatty acids = .7 g Omega-6 fatty acids = .6 g. Weight Watchers Winning Points = 5

❖ Preheat oven to 350°F. Line a 9 × 13 × 2-inch baking pan with a sheet of foil, wrapping excess up and around the outer edges of the pan. Coat bottom and sides of foil-lined pan with canola cooking spray.

❖ Add cake mix, canola oil, ¼ cup chocolate syrup, and ⅔ cup evaporated milk to mixing bowl and beat on medium-low speed for 1 minute. Scrape sides and stir in flaxseed.

❖ Spread batter evenly in prepared pan. Bake in center of oven for about 18 to 22 minutes or until center holds its shape but is still moist and slightly fudgy (test the center with a fork to be sure—do not overcook).

❖ Remove from oven and begin making frosting. Add 2 tablespoons butter, 3 tablespoons chocolate syrup, cocoa, and vanilla to small mixing bowl and beat on low until blended. Add powdered sugar and ¼ cup of milk and beat on low until smooth. Stir in the marshmallows and spread evenly over the top of the slightly warm brownies. Sprinkle walnuts over the top if desired. Let cool.

Pack a Punch Fruit Salad

MAKES 4 SERVINGS

৵

You can get 100 percent of many essential vitamins and minerals with just one serving of this juicy fruit salad.

4 cups assorted fresh (in season) summer fruit—ready to eat

2 tablespoons frozen "fruit punch" concentrate, thawed (cran-raspberry or similar concentrate can be substituted)

2 cups low-fat granola with raisins plus ¼ cup ground flaxseed (or use 2 cups of granola that contains ground flaxseed)

❖ Prepare each fruit for the salad (wash, cut, and pit apricots; wash, stem, and slice strawberries; wash seedless California grapes, etc.) and place in serving bowl.

❖ Drizzle thawed concentrated "fruit punch" juice over the top and toss to coat fruit well. Spoon into 4 bowls, sprinkle each with ½ cup of ground flaxseed containing granola, or low-fat granola that has been tossed with ground golden flaxseed, and enjoy.

NOTE: A 1-cup serving of this fruit salad gives you almost 100 percent of your recommended daily allowance for vitamin C, about a third of your recommended daily allowance for vitamin A, and 10 percent of your daily allowance for folic acid, vitamin B_6, vitamin E, and selenium.

PER SERVING (USING STRAWBERRIES AND PEACH SLICES): 276 calories, 6.2 g protein, 55 g carbohydrate, 5 g fat (.9 g saturated fat, 1.7 g monounsaturated fat, 2.5 g polyunsaturated fat) 0 mg cholesterol, 8.2 g fiber, 114 mg sodium. Calories from fat: 16 percent. Omega-3 fatty acids = 1.6 g Omega-6 fatty acids = .5 g. Weight Watchers Winning Points = 5

Kahlua Chocolate Fudge Cake

MAKES 12 SERVINGS

This cake is one of my favorites—and the dark color of the cake is a great disguise for the flaxseed.

Canola cooking spray

1 box Betty Crocker's Super Moist Devil's Food or Chocolate Fudge cake mix (or similar)

1 egg

2 egg whites (or ¼ cup egg substitute)

1 16-ounce container fat-free sour cream (light sour cream can be used)

¾ cup Kahlua or other coffee liqueur

¼ cup chocolate syrup

¾ cup ground flaxseed

Glaze:

⅔ cup white chocolate chips

2 tablespoons Kahlua or other coffee liqueur

Garnish:

1/4 cup semisweet mini or regular chocolate chips (optional)

❖ Preheat oven to 350°F. Coat the bottoms and sides of a bundt or tube pan generously with canola cooking spray.

❖ Add cake mix, egg, egg whites, sour cream, Kahlua, and chocolate syrup to mixing bowl. Beat on low for about 30 seconds. Scrape the bowl well and beat for another 30 seconds or until well blended. Stir in flaxseed.

❖ Spread batter into prepared cake pan, evening out top with a scraper. Bake about 45 minutes or until toothpick inserted into center comes out almost clean (this cake's texture is moister and more like a pudding cake than regular chocolate cake). Cool 10 minutes in pan. Cool cake completely and remove cake from pan before frosting.

❖ For glaze, add ⅔ cup white chocolate chips and 2 tablespoons Kahlua to microwave-safe glass measuring cup. Heat on HIGH 1 minute. Stir until chocolate chips are completely melted and blended with Kahlua to make a creamy glaze. Heat for 10 seconds or so. longer if needed. Drizzle or spread glaze over the top of cake.

Sprinkle mini chocolate chips over the glaze for extra garnish if desired. Store at room temperature.

NOTE: A serving of cake without glaze contains 342 calories, 9 grams fat, and 2.5 grams saturated fat.

PER SERVING (WITH GLAZE): 403 calories, 8 g protein, 59 g carbohydrate, 12 g fat (4.4 g saturated fat, 1.6 g monounsaturated fat, 2 g polyunsaturated fat), 50 mg cholesterol, 4 g fiber, 430 mg sodium. Calories from fat: 27 percent. Omega-3 fatty acids = 1.5 g Omega-6 fatty acids = .5 g. Weight Watchers Winning Points = 8

Any Fruit Flax Crisp

ॐ

You can design your own fruit crisp with this recipe—just decide which fruit to use in the filling. Better yet, you can combine two different fruits. My two favorite combinations are peach and raspberries and mango and boysenberries.

Crisp Topping:

⅓ cup walnuts

⅔ cup all-purpose flour

¼ cup ground flaxseed

3 tablespoons brown sugar

¼ teaspoon ground cinnamon

Pinch of salt (if using unsalted butter)

3 tablespoons butter, melted (in microwave or small saucepan)

3 tablespoons maple syrup, pancake syrup, or "lite" pancake syrup

Filling:

4 cups peeled and sliced or coarsely chopped fruit, or cut in a ½-inch dice*

¼ cup sugar

2 tablespoons flour (if fruit seems particularly juicy, increase this by a tablespoon)

*If using boysenberries, raspberries, blackberries, or blueberries, use whole—don't chop or slice. If using strawberries, cut into thick slices.

❖ Preheat oven to 375°F. Toast the walnuts by spreading on a pie plate and heating in oven until fragrant, about 7 minutes. Chop the nuts medium-fine.

❖ Combine the flour, flaxseed, brown sugar, cinnamon, and salt (if using unsalted butter) in a mixing bowl. Drizzle the melted butter and maple syrup over the top and blend on low speed until crumbly. Add the chopped nuts and mix well. The topping can be prepared up to a week ahead and refrigerated.

❖ Put the diced or sliced fruit in a large bowl. Add the sugar and taste; add more if necessary. Sprinkle the flour over the fruit and mix gently. Turn mixture into a 2-quart baking dish.

❖ Spoon the topping over the pears, pressing down lightly. Place the dish on a baking sheet (if necessary) to catch any overflow. Bake on the center rack of oven until the topping is golden brown and the juices have thickened slightly, about 35 to 45 minutes.

❖ Serve warm with light vanilla ice cream.

NOTE: If using sliced apples as filling or part of filling, you may only need to add 1 tablespoon of flour (if at all).

PER SERVING (WITH 2 CUPS RASPBERRIES AND 2 CUPS PEACH SLICES): 308 calories, 5 g protein, 48 g carbohydrate, 11.5 g fat (4 g saturated fat, 2.7 g monounsaturated fat, 4.7 g polyunsaturated fat), 15 mg cholesterol, 6.3 g fiber, 63 mg sodium. Calories from fat: 33 percent. Omega-3 fatty acids = 1.7 g Omega-6 fatty acids = 3 g. Weight Watchers Winning Points = 6

Key Lime Tart

MAKES 6 TO 8 TARTS

❧

Key lime pie is one of my favorite desserts so I was very motivated to try and come up with a way to work some flaxseed in. You may not even notice flaxseed is in this dessert—I discovered that when you mix ground flax with chopped nuts, it blends in quite nicely.

Filling:

1 envelope (scant tablespoon) unflavored gelatin

¼ cup water

1 14-ounce can fat-free sweetened condensed milk

½ cup egg substitute

4 ounces light or fat-free cream cheese

½ cup key lime juice (regular lime juice will work too)

Zest from 1 lime, finely chopped (optional)

Topping:

¼ cup macadamia nuts

3 tablespoons sweetened shredded coconut

3 tablespoons ground flaxseed

Light whipped cream or Cool Whip Free Whipped Topping (optional)

❖ Blend gelatin with water in small, nonstick saucepan and let sit for 1 minute. Cook over low heat, stirring constantly, until the gelatin dissolves and the mixture is clear (about 5 minutes). Set aside to cool.

❖ Place condensed milk, egg substitute, and cream cheese in food processor or blender. Pulse until combined. Slowly add the lime juice while the food processor is running. Blend an additional minute until mixture is nicely thickened. Gently pulse in gelatin mixture and lime zest (if desired). Pour or spoon into 6 to 8 custard cups (or similar)

❖ Add macadamia nuts, coconut, and flaxseed to small food processor (or hand chopper) and grind together briefly until nuts are just chopped. Sprinkle topping evenly over the key lime tarts. Cover with plastic wrap and refrigerate until set, about 2 hours. Serve each with a dollop of light whipped cream or Cool Whip if desired.

PER TART: 304 calories, 12 g protein, 46 g carbohydrates, 8 g fat (2.7 g saturated fat, 3.6 g monounsaturated fat, 1 g polyunsaturated fat), 11 mg cholesterol, 2 g fiber, 207 mg sodium. Calories from fat: 24 percent. Omega-3 fatty acids = .8 g Omega-6 fatty acids = .3 g. Weight Watchers Winning Points = 6

Raspberry Coconut Bars

MAKES 24 BARS

~

Don't confuse these with the more famous lemon bars. These bars have coconut and chopped pecans and are topped with a thin baked meringue– type topping.

Canola cooking spray

6 tablespoons butter, softened

6 tablespoons light cream cheese

1½ cups sugar

2 eggs, separated

1½ cups all-purpose flour

¾ cup raspberry reduced-sugar preserves (you can buy seedless or
regular preserves if you prefer)

⅓ cup ground golden flaxseed (golden
flax works best in this recipe)

½ cup shredded coconut

½ cup chopped pecans

❖ Preheat oven to 350°F. Coat a 13 × 9 × 2-inch baking pan with canola cooking spray.

❖ In electric mixer, beat the butter, cream cheese, and 1 cup of sugar until light and fluffy. Beat in egg yolks and gradually add the flour. Spread into prepared pan and bake for about 15 minutes.

❖ Meanwhile, add preserves to a 1-cup glass measure and warm in microwave (about 30 seconds on HIGH) until nice and loose. Stir in flaxseed. Cool bars slightly from the oven, then spread with raspberry preserve mixture; sprinkle with coconut.

❖ Beat egg whites until stiff. Gradually beat in the remaining ½ cup sugar until soft peaks form. Gently fold in the pecans. Spread mixture over the raspberry preserve layer and bake again at 350°F for 8 to 10 minutes or until top is lightly golden brown.

PER BAR: 160 calories, 2.5 g protein, 24 g carbohydrate, 6.5 g fat (3.2 g saturated fat, 2.2 g monounsatureted fat, 1.1 g polyunsaturated fat), 27 mg cholesterol, 1.5 g fiber, 61 mg sodium. Calories from fat: 38 percent. Omega-3 fatty acids = .4 g Omega-6 fatty acids = .7 g. Weight Watchers Winning Points = 3

Butterscotch Gingerbread Cookies

MAKES 32 LARGE COOKIES

❧

These chewy cookies just hit the spot, with their delicious combination of gingerbread spices and butterscotch chips.

2½ cups all-purpose flour

½ cup ground golden flaxseed (golden works best in this recipe)

2 teaspoons baking soda

1½ teaspoons ground cinnamon

1½ teaspoons ground ginger

¾ teaspoon ground cloves

½ teaspoon salt

10 tablespoons butter or canola margarine, softened

6 tablespoons honey

1 cup brown sugar, packed

1 large egg

⅓ cup light molasses

1½ cups butterscotch-flavored morsels (butterscotch chips)

❖ Preheat oven to 350°F.

❖ Combine flour, flaxseed, baking soda, cinnamon, ginger, cloves, and salt in small bowl.

❖ Beat butter, honey, brown sugar, egg, and molasses in large mixer bowl until fluffy and creamy. Gradually beat in flour mixture until well blended. Stir in butterscotch chips.

❖ Use cookie scoop to drop (2 tablespoons of cookie dough) dough onto baking sheets that have been coated with canola cooking spray. Press dough down with fingers or palms to lightly flatten.

❖ Bake for about 10 minutes or until cookies are lightly browned but still soft. Remove to wire racks to cool completely.

PER LARGE COOKIE: 160 calories, 1.8 g protein, 25 g carbohydrate, 6 g fat (4 g saturated fat, 1.4 g monounsaturated fat, .6 g polyunsaturated fat), 16 mg cholesterol, 1.5 g fiber, 165 mg sodium. Calories from fat: 36 percent. Omega-3 fatty acids = .4 g Omega-6 fatty acids = .2 g. Weight Watchers Winning Points = 3

Acknowledgments

Truly, this book would not be possible without the dedicated people who have conducted research on flaxseed over the past decade. Many have been relentless in their pursuit of understanding the benefits and physiological effects of flax. I am not a researcher; I am a registered dietitian who happens to write books and magazine articles on health and nutrition—so I would be nowhere without the hard work of these researchers. Thanks to them I have lots of exciting information to share with you! A special thank-you to one of the first flaxseed researchers, Lilian Thompson from the University of Toronto, who continues to amaze me with all of her accomplishments and who so generously answered several of my question-filled emails. Lastly, I am eternally grateful to Steven Cunane, also a flax researcher with the University of Toronto, who took time out of his busy schedule to review the not-so-brief chapter 1 for me.

Notes

Page 10, Mantzioris et al., Rheumatology Unit of the Royal Adelaide Hospital in Australia: "Eat a higher omega-3 diet for two weeks and . . .," *American Journal of Clinical Nutrition,* July 2000, 72(1):42-48.

Page 19, "Recently the American Dietetic Association (ADA) published . . .," *Journal of the American Dietetic Association,* July 2002, 102(7):993–1000.

Page 21, Howe et al.: "Recently the results of 13 case-control studies on diet . . .," *Journal of the National Cancer Institute,* 1992, 84:1887–1896.

Page 21, Howe et al.: "When researchers pooled the results of twelve case-control studies . . .," *Journal of the National Cancer Institute,* 1990, 82:561–569.

Page 21, "Caution—All fiber intake recommendations need to recognize . . .," JADA—Position Paper on the Health Implications of Dietary Fiber

Page 23, Thompson et al.: "Tumor size was lower in the rats . . .," *Carcinogenesis,* 1996, 17:1373–1376.

Page 23, Jenab and Thompson: "Flaxseed rat studies have also demonstrated . . .," *Carcinogenesis,* 1996, 17:1343–1348.

Page 23, "After testing the effect of just lignans on human colon tumor cell lines . . .," *Anticancer Research,* May–June 1998, 18(3A):1405–1408.

Page 23, "Dr. Demark-Wahnefried of Duke University Medical Center . . .," *Anticancer Research,* 2001, 21:3995–4000.

Page 24, Thompson et al.: "And guess what happened—the researchers found tumor growth reduced . . .," *Abstract Preview: BCSOL_157 "Biological Effects of Dietary Flaxseed in Patients with Breast Cancer."* Nutritional Sciences, University of Toronto.

Page 25, "For example, a recent study concluded that phytoestrogens . . .," *American Journal of Clinical Nutrition,* September 2000, 72(3):844–852.

Page 26, "The lignans in flaxseed appear to be . . .," *Carcinogenesis*, June 1996, 17(6):1373–1376.

Page 27, Thompson et al.: "They concluded that while the lignans in flaxseed appear . . .," *Carcinogenesis*, June 1996, 17(6):1373–1376. Department of Nutritional Sciences, University of Toronto.

Page 27, "Dr. Slavin suggests that since previous studies show . . .," *Nutr Cancer* 2001, 39(1):58-65; this study was also presented at the 222nd national meeting of the American Chemical Society.

Page 28, Demark-Wahnefried et al.: "Dr. Demark-Wahnefried has already begun . . .," *Urology*, July 2001, 58:47–52. Duke University Medical Center.

Page 29, "The lignan-treated group not only . . .," *Cancer Letter*, Jul 19, 1999, 142(1):91–96.

Page 30, Cunnane et al.: "The levels of omega-3s increased . . .," *American Journal of Clinical Nutrition*, January 1995, 61(1):62–68. Department of Nutritional Sciences, University of Toronto.

Page 30, "The oxidation of LDLs is thought to . . .," *Archives of Internal Medicine*, 1999, 159:1313–1320.

Page 31, Prasad: "But flaxseed did this without significantly . . .," *Atherosclerosis*, Jul 11, 1997, 132(1):69–76. Department of Physiology, University of Saskatchewan, Canada.

Page 31, "The omega-3s have exhibited antiarrhythmic effects . . .," *Lancet*, 1999, 354:447–455.

Page 31, "They may be doing this by modifying . . .," *Journal of Nutrition*, 1997, 127:383–393.

Page 31, "The flaxseed decreased total cholesterol . . .," press release from the American Physiological Society, April 23, 2002.

Page 32, "One study, which found that as the plant . . .," *Stroke*, 1995, 26:778–782.

Page 32, Simopoulos: "Fish oil, a particularly potent source of omega-3s, has . . .," *Canadian Journal of Physiological Pharmacolology*, March 1997, 75(3):234–239. Center for Genetics, Nutrition and Health.

Page 33, "By day 101 . . .," *Journal of Laboratory Clinical Medicine*, July 2001, 138(1):32–39.

Page 33, Cunnane et al.: "One study of healthy young adults found that . . .," *American Journal of Clinical Nutrition*, January 1995, 61(1):62–68. Department of Nutritional Sciences, University of Toronto.

Page 34, "The patients consumed 15 to 45 grams of flaxseed . . .," *Kidney Int.*, 1995, 48:475–480.

Page 35, James and Cleland. "Increasing omega-3s and decreasing . . .," *Semin Arthritis Rheum*, October 1997, 27(2):85–97. Rheumatology.

Page 36, "Other studies have also suggested that . . .," *British Medical Journal*, 1996, 313:84–90; and *American Journal of Clinical Nutrition*, 1999, 69:890–897.

Page 36, Mantzioris et al.: "But when we eat fish . . .," *American Journal of Clinical Nutrition*, July 2000, 72(1):42–48.

Page 53, *J Agric Food Chem*, March 13, 2002, 50(6):1668–1671.

Index